MUSCLES AND MERIDIANS

For Elsevier
Publisher: Sarena Wolfaard
Development Editor: Sheila Black
Project Manager: Joannah Duncan
Design Direction: Stewart Larking
Illustration Manager: Gillian Richards
Illustrator: Graeme Chambers

MUSCLES AND MERIDIANS

THE MANIPULATION OF SHAPE

Phillip Beach DO DAc OSNZ
Osteopathic and Acupunture Practitioner
Wellington
New Zealand

Foreword by
Leon Chaitow ND DO
Registered Osteopath and Naturopath;
Honorary Fellow and Former Senior Lecturer,
School of Life Sciences, University of Westminster,
London, UK;
Fellow, British Naturopathic Association

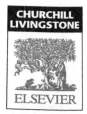

EDINBURGH LONDON NEW YORK OXFORD PHILADELPHIA ST LOUIS
SYDNEY TORONTO 2010

CHURCHILL
LIVINGSTONE
ELSEVIER

© 2010 Elsevier Ltd. All rights reserved.

ISBN 978-0-7020-3109-0

British Library Cataloguing in Publication Data
A catalogue record for this book is available from the British Library

Library of Congress Cataloging in Publication Data
A catalog record for this book is available from the Library of Congress

Notices
Knowledge and best practice in this field are constantly changing. As new research and experience broaden our understanding, changes in research methods, professional practices, or medical treatment may become necessary.

Practitioners and researchers must always rely on their own experience and knowledge in evaluating and using any information, methods, compounds, or experiments described herein. In using such information or methods they should be mindful of their own safety and the safety of others, including parties for whom they have a professional responsibility.

With respect to any drug or pharmaceutical products identified, readers are advised to check the most current information provided (i) on procedures featured or (ii) by the manufacturer of each product to be administered, to verify the recommended dose or formula, the method and duration of administration, and contraindications. It is the responsibility of practitioners, relying on their own experience and knowledge of their patients, to make diagnoses, to determine dosages and the best treatment for each individual patient, and to take all appropriate safety precautions.

To the fullest extent of the law, neither the Publisher nor the authors, contributors, or editors, assume any liability for any injury and/or damage to persons or property as a matter of products liability, negligence or otherwise, or from any use or operation of any methods, products, instructions, or ideas contained in the Material herein.

Printed in China

CONTENTS

FOREWORD

Clarity is slowly emerging, from various disciplines, regarding the complexly integrated way the body functions. Recent research by scientists such as Ingber (2006), Langevin et al (2001), and Schleip et al (2005), as well as clinicians and anatomists such as Hedley (2007), Stecco (2007), and Myers (2009), has helped to reveal more clearly – for example – the important role of fascial structures in offering shape, coherence, stability, mobility, and communication potential to the body's economy.

Another part of that understanding involves a greater appreciation of the importance of tensegrity in the architecture of everything, from the cell to gross human musculo-ligamento-skeletal structures – and how they move and function. Equally this growing understanding of the interconnectedness of everything helps to clarify why restriction, dysfunction, and tissue modification (resulting from pathology, overuse, misuse, abuse, or disuse) in one part of the body can produce major repercussions at a distance.

As two recent Fascia Research congresses have made clear (Boston 2007, Amsterdam 2009), much remains to be revealed as these concepts are studied, both by research scientists and clinicians. By looking backward in time into the very origins of life, as well as by close observation of his patients, and via a series of remarkable insights, Phillip Beach has performed the heroic task of moving our understanding further.

By surveying, investigating, and charting the human condition relative to shape, posture, and movement (he describes movement as 'the coherent changing of shape') – in the contexts of evolution (how did early life forms move?), embryology (the extraordinary processes of cleavage, folding, compaction, and more of the embryonic disc, to the point where limb buds, arches, and the beginnings of sense organs appear), childhood development, physiology, and neural function, and what he terms 'archetypal postures' – Phillip Beach has advanced our understanding and has offered a new way of understanding the way the human body works – or fails to work when unbalanced and out of synchronization ('out of tune') with its optimal patterns.

Beach's training in osteopathic medicine, his exploration of dance, martial arts, movement therapies (such as Pilates and yoga), and his understanding of Traditional Chinese Medicine's (TCM) meridian maps, have informed his investigations and findings – for example of movement patterns that he terms 'contractile fields', which are structurally and functionally connected to sense organs. In building the arguments for the validity of his findings he notes a neurological hierarchy, in which the organs of sense, taste, sight, smell, etc.

offer the cues that drive much basic, primitive, movement. He also focuses attention on the adaptive processes involved in our anti-gravity evolutionary struggle to rise from the floor – where sitting, squatting, crawling, and wriggling are more appropriate – to the upright where standing and walking become possible.

The way in which his enlightened insights move from the likelihood that evolutionary and developmental patterns of movement may be strongly associated with organs of sense, to the idea that these very movements, or the contractile elements associated with them, determine the shape and connections that are described as TCM's acupuncture meridians, is both thought-provoking and therapeutically exciting.

One way of viewing much musculoskeletal pain and dysfunction is as failed adaptation. What Beach has done is to paint a very big canvas indeed, where adaptation takes on a wider meaning than is commonly conceived – and where potential clinical solutions lie in a greater understanding of these themes emerging from a background of evolution, embryology, and patterns of contractility, that may be assessed and modified via appropriate therapeutic interventions.

Among the common-sense approaches suggested by this detailed exploration of the body are some extremely simple and clinically practical suggestions:

- To spend more time on the floor in 'archetypal postures of repose' such as squatting, kneeling, cross-legged, tailor's position, and long sitting
- To revisit the processes involved in rising from the floor to upright
- To pay attention to the state of our feet (Beach rails repeatedly against shoes, which he describes as 'sensory deprivation chambers').

Beach acknowledges that: 'Because of the exploratory nature of the book, aspects of the work will prove to be too speculative, for which I take responsibility.' However, this should not detract from the potential clinical value of the broad ideas that emerge in this book.

I for one have learnt a great deal from the ideas explored and synthesized – and believe that the book will take its place as the cornerstone of a branch of manual therapy that detaches itself from modalities, and historical professional allegiances, offering as it does both explanations and new therapeutic directions.

Leon Chaitow ND DO

REFERENCES

Hedley G 2007 Demonstration of the integrity of human superficial fascia as an autonomous organ. In: Findley T, Schleip R (eds) Fascia research: basic science and implications for conventional and complementary health care. Elsevier Urban and Fischer, Munich, pp 134–135

Ingber DE 2006 Cellular mechanotransduction: putting all the pieces together again. Journal of the Federation of American Societies for Experimental Biology 20:811–827

Langevin HM, Churchill DL, Cipolla MJ 2001 Mechanical signaling through connective tissue: a mechanism for the therapeutic effect of acupuncture. FASEB Journal 15:2275–2282

Myers T 2009 Anatomy trains: myofascial meridians for manual and movement therapists. Churchill Livingstone, Edinburgh

Schleip R, Klinger W, Lehmann F 2005
Active fascial contractility: fascia may be
able to contract in a smooth muscle-like
manner and thereby influence
musculoskeletal dynamics. Medical
Hypotheses 65:273–277

Stecco C 2007 Histological study of deep
fasciae of the limbs. In: Findley T, Schleip
R (eds) Fascia research: basic science and
implications for conventional and
complementary health care. Elsevier
Urban and Fischer, Munich, pp 132–133

Foreword

PREFACE

Our shape preoccupies us all. Are we in good shape, bad shape, or do we just need to shape up? We also move by changing our shape. For example, walking and running are rhythmic changes of body shape. The manipulation of human shape is tackled from three perspectives in this book. The book explores the question 'are there patterns we can discern that are common to, or underlie, how we change shape?'

Those patterns must emerge from behaviours that vertebrates have employed during a half a billion year time frame. Fish bend side to side, dolphins bend up and down, and humans contra-twist their shoulders and hips to walk, run, and throw. These are primal patterns that are embedded in our physiques. Each of these primary patterns of movement I call a contractile field. The fields are a structural and functional synthesis of many anatomical tissues, but the contractile field model stresses that it is the interaction of the fields that creates coherent shape change.

Are some shapes more important than others, and, if so, why are those shapes deemed important? The opposite of animal movement is the resting state or shape of an organism. Rest is to movement as night is to day. Considering movement without concurrently considering rest is illogical. Postures that all humankind has rested in for millions of years are important not just to rest but also to the movement that ensues. This book suggests that, as a society, we need to place a new value on the postures we need to rest in, described in this context as 'archetypal postures of repose.' Each posture is a developmental birthright that helps 'tune' our hundreds of named muscles and joints towards deeply embedded preferred shapes.

The meridians of Traditional Chinese Medicine are used by acupuncturists around the world when they treat patients. Meridians are lines on the body that the Chinese mapped 2000+ years ago. What did the Chinese have in mind when they mapped the body with these enigmatic lines? When I was a student of acupuncture, the meridial map was presented to me as a received wisdom that we needed to rote learn. Using both the contractile field model and the archetypal postures a new 'decoding' of the meridial map is proposed. The number, location, pairing, and networking of the meridians takes on a cohesive meaning. I have a new respect for what the Chinese medical theorists were grappling with so long ago.

The book has evolved as one idea opened the door to another. Sometimes the link from one insight to the next was like a breathless cascade whilst at other times the development of the ideas struck an obstacle that I could not see past. Due to the exploratory nature of this book, aspects of the work will prove to be too speculative, for which I take responsibility. However, by trying to conform to the evolution and embryology of our species the process tends to be self-corrective as these are the larger truths that underlie our existence.

Many people have contributed to the development of these ideas. Serge Gracovetsky changed the way I thought about biomechanics. Professor Brian Goodwin helped me look at science in a less compartmentalized manner. Phillip Silverman has been a real help in the writing process, as has Sheila Black from Elsevier, who gently kept me on track. In particular, I would like to thank Inge Cordsen, John Beach, Edward Posey, and Robyn Pearce, who have offered me their trust and support.

Phillip Beach
Wellington, 2010

Introduction

A patient presented to my clinic in Wellington, New Zealand complaining of low back pain, left buttock pain, chronic tension with episodic pain across both shoulders/neck, and almost as an afterthought, discomfort with 'noises' from both knees. This pleasant woman was in her middle 40s, worked at a desk, was about 15 kg overweight, and found the 1 km walk to my practice hard work. Where does one start when attempting to address her various complaints?

This type of presentation is all too common. Diffuse musculoskeletal distress (also known as regional pain syndromes) appears to be endemic within our society. People of all hues seem to be afflicted. It is hard to discern underlying patterns when both male and female, young and old, fit and unfit, stiff and flexible, thin and fat are affected – dichotomies of many shades but similarly afflicted by chronic musculoskeletal dis-ease that periodically flares up. The personal cost and the cost to society is simply staggering.

A whole gamut of professions and research avenues are called upon to address these disorders of movement, but with little consensus yet to emerge as to a common conceptual understanding (Kent et al 2009). It appears we need to revise aspects of our understanding of the neuromusculoskeletal system that moves us and is the source of so much of this type of everyday dis-ease. Below I will introduce a new model of human movement (the 'contractile field' model) that is then developed in later chapters. Crucial to treatment is assessment – a new model of movement engenders a different approach to assessment; a methodology called the 'archetypal postures' is proposed. Simple assessment procedures will be introduced that look for the 'tune' of the musculoskeletal system. The word 'tune' implies proper for purpose, harmony, accord, with music often a reference context. Tune as used here is the harmonious interaction of thousands of named anatomical structures. Watching a person walking effortlessly compared with a person walking with osteoarthritis of a hip joint gives us a sense of tune that is like a summative insight into the ease or otherwise of that movement pattern. As in music, tune can be reduced to reference notes that I suggest in this context are the archetypal postures. In the author's experience, patients quickly grasp the implications of being 'in or out of tune', and find the treatment and advice offered easy to comprehend and comply with. These ideas are then used to consider the meridians of Traditional Chinese Medicine (TCM), the final chapters of the book. Thus the three primary themes that form the warp and weft of this book are movement, archetypal postures, and meridians.

1

The first theme concerns the awe-inspiring complexity of human movement. From 1979 to 1983 I studied osteopathy at the British College of Osteopathic Medicine in London. As an undergraduate I was interested in how multiple muscles might functionally link together to move the body, an idea that was then called 'muscle chains.' Traditional musculoskeletal anatomy is taught bone-by-bone, joint-by-joint, and muscle-by-muscle. Each structure is carefully revealed by the painstaking dissection of a cadaver. Obviously, cadavers do not move, nor do they complain – quite unlike the patients I treated at the college clinic! My fourth-year thesis revolved around the topic of dance injury. I collated what little there was then in the academic literature, and supplemented this with interviews of dancers at the Laban School of Dance (London), Alan Herdman (Pilates), and teachers from the yoga/martial arts world. I soon realized my cadaver-based anatomical studies gave me little insight into how power and poise were derived from the underlying muscle matrix.

My enquiry into the nature of whole person movement patterns took on a new momentum when I read *Bright Air, Brilliant Fire* by Gerald Edelman (1992), a book that looks at how Darwinian concepts can be applied to neurology. Of interest to me was the context Edelman suggested was needed to approach something as complex as brain and mind. Only a synthesis derived from a knowledge of the evolution of animal nervous systems, the embryological/childhood development of the nervous system, allied with anatomy/physiology would get close to understanding something as complex as brain and mind. Edelman's approach appealed to me so I then decided to employ a similar broad scope in my enquiry of human movement.

I have developed an understanding of human movement that I call the 'contractile field' (CF) model. The word 'contractile' was selected as I did not want to define the concept by a named anatomical tissue. Individual cells have contractile elements, and tissue not usually associated with movement, such as fascia, has demonstrated contractility (Schleip et al 2005). As we shall see, the CF model suggests that both blood pressure and kidney function profoundly affect our movement patterns. Fields are defined as an area of operation, a region in which some common condition prevails. The CF model explores the innate patterning found in the human neuromuscular system. Based on an analysis of vertebrate movement, I have identified the minimum number of interactive CFs needed for primary human movement patterns. Each of the proposed CFs will be described in terms of its evolutionary and embryological derivation. The fields will have their borders delineated, and field interpenetration will be considered.

Dissective anatomy teaches us that a nerve from the brain or spinal cord innervates every voluntary muscle, an association that is so close, the two systems are commonly linked together as a 'neuromuscular system.' When a CF is described – a field of contractility that spans head to tail – its innervation would span from the cranial region to the coccygeal region. Each CF would be similarly innervated, and thus a meaningless association in this whole person context.

What is needed for a whole field of contractility is a supra-segmental form of innervation. In the neurological hierarchy, the primary sense organs are profoundly important to any animal as they inform and direct movement. Where it is appropriate, the CF is modelled as embedding a sense organ, a novel association suggested to me via the Chinese meridial map.

Like models for weather or climate change, the CF model is not a definitive mapping of the muscle matrix. Rather it is a starting point that will foster the development of this modelling process. However, modelling human movement in terms of interacting fields of contractility is of real use to all those professions that attend the moving body. It is an idea whose time has come.

ARCHETYPAL POSTURES

A new way of looking at musculoskeletal anatomy and function will encourage and inform a new approach to an assessment methodology, the second major theme of this book. CFs model movement. The opposite of animal movement is animal rest – movement and rest are flip sides of the same coin. One without the other is nonsensical. When I examine a new patient I ask them to assume a number of postures – 'archetypal postures of repose.' These include lying on one's back, lying on the front, sitting cross-legged, kneeling Japanese style, and squatting. Each of these postures has an evolutionary history that goes back to our common ancestor with the other apes millions of years ago. I suggest modern lifestyles have divorced us from a natural form of biomechanical self-correction with a resultant back pain that has become endemic in our societies.

Sitting on the floor in comfort is a developmental birthright. Every young child on this planet masters floor sitting postures as a precursor to standing, walking and running. From floor sitting to then erect from the floor is a profound movement pattern. It uses hundreds of named muscles to lift many kilos from the floor upward. It is the anti-gravity exercise. A floor living lifestyle, without further ado, means erecting from the floor many times a day. I have developed a series of exercises called the 'Erectorcise' as a way of maintaining this crucial series of movements. The Erectorcise exercises are all derived from the many ways we can erect from the floor.

Archetypal postures and erecting oneself from the floor are two legs of a clinically applicable tripod of ideas. The third idea is the crucial role our feet play in our biomechanical well-being. Standing up on hind limbs initiated a cascade of evolutionary metamorphosis that has affected every aspect of our being. But at a cost. Four living support platforms are reduced to just two. We then cover the two feet with thick leather or man-made mush that reduce the crucial raw data input a now precariously balanced upright body needs in order to move with power and poise. I call shoes sensory deprivation chambers that blind our low back in particular. Rehabilitating our feet is essential if we are to help reduce the incidence and severity of musculoskeletal distress, and our tendency to fall over as we get older.

It is the author's opinion that one cannot understand clinical human biomechanics without an appreciation of these fundamental body postures and the importance of the feet to musculoskeletal health. Archetypal postures, and the effort to erect oneself from the floor to standing are a way of fine-tuning the many muscles we use in life. Biomechanical tune is an emergent property that can be assessed. The concept of musculoskeletal tune is not the

Introduction

3

icing on a biomechanical cake, rather it is as crucial, as non-negotiable, as tune is to a musical instrument.

MERIDIANS

The third broad theme of the book concerns the meridians of Chinese medicine. In the late 1980s I studied Traditional Chinese Medicine (TCM) as I suspected a stretching of my conceptual frameworks would be helpful. Osteopathy is grounded in a biomedical model of the body, with lip service paid to a whole person approach to diagnosis and treatment. Was there another perspective? Chinese medical theorists more than 2000 years ago, after profound study, mapped what they perceived to be the flow of Blood and Qi within conduits that we will call meridians. Use of this map via manual therapy, needles, cauterization, and exercises still forms the basis of the acu-moxa branch of TCM.

The meridial map is extremely detailed. A recent Western text on meridians/acupoints runs to more than 600 pages, describing in scrupulous anatomical detail the meridians and acupoints (Deadman et al 1998). Fourteen named meridians run up and down the torso. The arm has six meridians in a regular pattern whereas the six leg meridians are crossed and generally more complex. On meridians are acupoints that are said to predictably influence visceral function. For example, Lung-7 (Lieque) near the ventral/lateral wrist is a main point on the body for many lung organ dysfunctions.

However, the map has problems from a bioscientific perspective. Scanning electron microscopy, microscopic dissection, thermal imaging, radioactive tagging techniques, magnetic resonance imaging (MRI) and positron emission tomography (PET) scans, etc. have all failed to find the meridians. Imagine that I point to an alcove and describe a small man that I shall call a hobbit; the 600-page description of this man I give is detailed, richly textured and nuanced. But you look, your friends look, photographs are taken, the alcove is carefully examined using microscopes, thermal and radioactive scanners, etc. and ... they all see nothing. In this respect, one of us is seemingly delusional. In the case of the meridial map, a whole culture, thousands of human years, hundreds of texts, have been describing something. A lot of prestige and cultural ego is on the line. But here we also have something remarkable. A well-preserved pre-scientific-era medical map that now is in worldwide clinical use. Acupuncture treatment is available to billions of people worldwide.

Firstly, what are meridians – what was being mapped over 2000 years ago? Chinese medical theory states that Qi and Blood flow in meridians was mapped. The cardiovascular system has been extensively studied over the last 350 years – meridians do not map blood vessels. Qi is an amorphous concept and the meridians it is purported to flow in have not been identified.

Secondly, how does an acupoint such as Lung-7 (Lieque) affect lung function, and do so predictably? From a biomedical viewpoint, this is nonsense. No lung tissue is in the arm for a starter. As a student of acupuncture one learns by rote and places trust in the Chinese seers of long ago. The meridial map certainly represents a profound and sustained cultural enquiry, but again, what did they map?

Bioscience has no answers to these questions. Without a working explanatory model the entire practice is seen as a belief system that probably relies on the placebo effect (and endogenous opiates) for much of its therapeutic effect. This is harsh, but understandable, if one has not invested years cloaked in the richness of image and metaphor that TCM can provide.

I have come to understand the meridians of TCM as 'emergent lines of shape control.' It is a deceptively simple phrase. The term 'acu-moxa' is shorthand for acupuncture and the burning of mugwort on or near the skin – both practices can elicit a basic survival reflex, i.e. recoil from a noxious stimulus. When something hurts you, such as a skin prick or burn, you recoil away. With the onset of predation via tooth, claw, and sting 500+ million years ago, recoil from hurt has had a long time to deeply embed itself in the way vertebrates wire their nervous and muscular systems together. There is a pattern to this recoil and I suggest the Chinese discerned and mapped key aspects of this pattern.

Here is the link between contractile fields and meridians. With the contractile field model of movement I could see how a pinprick would elicit a whole body movement. Lines (i.e. meridians) then emerge on the living body that, when pricked or pressed, will elicit the same basic movement pattern. As meridians are emergent from the whole living form they will not be found on a cadaver. In essence, I think the Chinese learnt to predictably influence subtle body shape by using a three-dimensional pattern of pinpricks. Shape and function dance closely together.

A thought experiment will be employed to flesh out the idea. Much of the arcane detail found in the meridial map becomes understandable, rational, and precocious, considering how many modern texts I have had to assimilate to come to terms with what I now propose was mapped. I have developed a new respect for the Traditional Chinese Medical map, and suggest it still has value today.

This book is directed toward all those who deal with the moving human body, its ease and its loss of ease. The first chapters step back to look at the big picture via deep time – the origin of moving animals, and back in personal time – our embryological development. Necessarily, this is a quick scan with only a few key aspects dwelled upon, but context is created. Then a chapter will draw together ideas that inform the modelling process, followed by chapters that will introduce each CF. It is the seamless interaction of CFs that shape human movement.

The concept of archetypal postures and biomechanical tune will be presented as an assessment methodology. If we are to make headway in reducing Western society's endemic musculoskeletal pain, new perspectives are needed. Surprisingly simple advice can have a profound effect on form and function.

Good modelling is often able to cross genre and, in this case, the CF model is employed to suggest a decoding of the Chinese meridial map. By decoding I mean to explain why the Chinese settled on 14 primary meridians, why they are classified and related as they are, what the Chinese were hinting at with the 'deep meridians,' and how they then mapped the acupoints. I do not argue for the efficacy of acupuncture, as in the modern world of evidence-based medicine, the practice will need to prove itself. Insight into what the

Chinese mapped will aid the transfer of a traditional medical practice to a new worldwide audience.

This book is not a technique manual, rather it offers context and explanation for all professions that have as a mandate the movement patterns found in a whole living person. Re-establishing powerful self-corrective mechanisms in our patients makes treating musculoskeletal distress more comprehensible and effective, whatever the modality used.

REFERENCES

Deadman P, Al-Khafaji M, Baker K 1998 A manual of acupuncture. Journal of Chinese Medicine Publications, Hove

Edelman G 1992 Bright air, brilliant fire. Penguin, London

Kent P, Keating J, Buchbinder R 2009 Searching for a conceptual framework for nonspecific low back pain. Manual Therapy 14(4):387–396

Schleip R, Klingler W, Lehmann-Horn F 2005 Active fascial contractility: fascia may be able to contract in a smooth muscle-like manner and thereby influence musculoskeletal dynamics. Medical Hypotheses 65:273–277

Muscles and meridians

6

A wriggle in deep time

I

CHAPTER CONTENTS

Animal life is constructed around robust operating systems called body-plans. Body-plans were established half a billion years ago and are still discernable today. The concept of body-plans focuses one's attention on what is really important in the construction of an animal.

This chapter will introduce the concept of body-plans. To model how we move our bodies it is first appropriate to look at bodies with the widest possible lens. A body-plan sets parameters to which all subsequent evolutionary development of that phylum must refer. All animals move by manipulating their shape; that shape has fundamental constructional rules that must be adhered to. All vertebrates have a sensory platform at the anterior pole of the animal, with sensory capsules devoted to olfaction, vision, and balance/ sound (distant touch). The brain and the sensory platform are wired together so that vertebrate cranial nerves across hundreds of millions of years show a similar topological layout.

Microbial life took an early and tenacious hold on this planet somewhere between 3.5 and 3.8 billion years ago. The search for the last universal common ancestor (the mythic LUCA) has spawned many rival theories. Rather than a heroic single act, the LUCA was probably a common ancestral community of gene-swapping primitive viruses and early cells (Hamilton 2005, 2008). For an unimaginable length of time, descendants of these cells, such as blue-green slime, clung to wet rock whilst microbial mats and

7

© 2010 Elsevier Ltd / Inc / Bv
DOI: 10.1016/B978-0-7020-3109-0.00006-7

fronds of algae floated on the seas under harsh light and extreme environmental conditions. Developing a bilaminar membrane that mediated transport across the cell boundary was a crucial innovation needed by cellular life. About 7 billion years ago (all these dates are loosely defined) multicellular animals emerged, primitive animals with no blood, gut tube or nervous system.

Ediacarans (ee-dee-ACK-rins) are an enigmatic group of animals, dated to 575–542 million years ago (MYA) that formed protoplasmic lumps within slime mats. Some types evolved an internally quilted or vaned appearance; others fossilized into complexly filigreed branching or spiralled structures. Ediacarans must have been peaceful neighbours of the microbial mats as they have left little evidence in the fossil record of offensive capacity. However, Life that had been unicellular for billions of years, Garden-of-Eden-like, started becoming more complex, but far more dangerous.

Between 542 and 489 MYA, in what is called the Cambrian explosion, larger multicellular animals with a bewildering array of body-plans emerged. 'Small shelly fossils' characterizing rocks from all over the world date from this time window (McMenamin & McMenamin 1990). They rapidly diversified into a riot of complexly shaped and colored animals that were on the move (McMenamin & McMenamin 1990).

The important word here is 'move.' To move is a profound act that started an innovation cascade. Aquatic animals 'learnt' how to move via a manipulation of their shape, with or against the substrate – the water or mud that enveloped them. Moving facilitated an exploration of the environment in the search for food. Interaction between animal and environment became increasingly complex.

During the Cambrian explosion of animal diversity it has been estimated that many body-plans emerged. A body-plan (also known as Baupläne) represents the rootstock, in a sense the archetype of that lineage of animal. All contemporary animal life on Earth coalesces down to about 35–38 fundamental body-plans, corresponding roughly to the phyla level of classification. Zoology discerns phyla using comparative morphology (shape and structure), physiology, shared patterns of embryological development, and insights derived from molecular biology. The Cambrian and the period following it display a cathartic exuberance of new animal phyla that experimented with complex bodies – an era of extraordinary, never to be repeated, innovation. Shells, brains, eyes, color, guts, and limbs all configured in ways that were unimaginable until fossils were found. All the major body-plans are marine in origin and were established by the close of the Cambrian period. Only one phylum level body-plan (the bryozoan) has arisen in the animal kingdom in the last 500 million years (Arthur 1997), in contrast to the plant kingdom where the flowering plants' body-plan arose relatively recently.

The initial exuberance of animal life was both pruned and re-stocked over the next 50 million years, but only 35–38 body-plans have survived those tumultuous times. Those that survived appear to be extraordinarily resilient. Even the Permian mass extinction (about 250 MYA), that most massive wipe-out of life on earth, with its spectacular decimation of marine animals to about 5% of their earlier diversity, shows no fossil evidence of new phyla in the re-radiation of animal life. Likewise, the colonization of land, a rich new environment, produced no new body-plans, in spite of the challenges imposed by gravity and dryness. Only seven animal phyla evolved adaptations allowing them full terrestrial lives above the soil surface (Raff 1996).

There must have been extraordinary ecological pressures to drive such a rapid flowering of diversity. A number of ideas have been postulated to explain why this proliferation of different animal phyla took place. Prior to the Cambrian, in the period 750–580 MYA, the Earth's climate was wild. Paleoclimatologists have identified a series of near whole planet glaciations rapidly followed by extreme heating. Massive sheets of ice migrated toward the equator followed by polar ice-cap meltdowns. Life's early hold was battered by climate, volcanism, and extraterrestrial impacts. About 535 MYA, the Earth's continental plates began an earth-wrenching migration – in 15 million years, continents vaulted through 90 degrees of latitude. Polar continents migrated to the equator and vice versa, tearing up the sea floor and again radically altering climate. Pre-Cambrian life was thus ecologically pulverized and radically disseminated, as climate change has always been a prime driver of evolution.

Life responded by developing a new type of body based on three, rather than two, embryonic cell layers. The new third layer is called mesoderm, a layer sandwiched between the two older layers that are called ectoderm and endoderm (Raff 1996). Mesoderm produces tissues that facilitate movement, both of fluids and food within the body, and to move the body in the environment. Movement creates choice – the whole point to movement involves an appraisal of the environment so that bio-rich pathways can be followed. Movement toward food, fellow, and comfort is still the way of the world. The early vertebrate brain was partitioned to specialize in the three types of incoming sensory data: chemical (smell and taste), electromagnetic (light and electric/magnetic fields), and movement (sound and touch). Movement directed by sense organs allowed a new way of life, the consequences of which we still face today. Long-range sensory detectors such as olfaction and vision, allied with close-range weapons – tooth and claw – suddenly turned on an arms race that we animals still participate in today. The first casualties in all this upheaval were the Ediacarans and the slime world. They disappeared from the fossil record during the pre-Cambrian, probably as fodder, a minority possibly evolving into the ancestor of some existent phyla.

To delineate one body-plan from another, crucial constructional features are looked for. Each body-plan has a suite of characteristics that interlock to produce a biological operating system of profound robustness; think Mac or Windows but with 500 million years of operational stability! Table 1.1 shows some essential building blocks that unite to form a body-plan.

Each of the character states will be introduced now as these ideas will be needed and aspects expanded upon in the following chapters. Imagine you are examining a new animal that has been found near a deep-sea vent or in an isolated forest in Vietnam. Your assessment would be based on the animal's external form – its morphology regarding size, shape, weight, and movement pattern. Dissection would reveal more information about how the internal anatomical structure is divided by body cavities and segmentation. The embryological genesis of that animal's form, an arcane study, would

Table 1.1 Some essential building blocks making up a body-plan (From Arthur 1997)	
Character states	Main character
Skeleton	Hydrostatic, internal, external
Symmetry	Bilateral, radial, asymmetric
Pairs of appendages	0, 2, 3, 4, many
Cleavage pattern	Meroblastic, holoblastic
Body cavity	Acoel, pseudocoel, coelom
Segmentation	Segmented, unsegmented

reveal much about the animal's developmental modus operandi, and by inference, its relationship to all animal development. By assessing the new animal in terms of the above chart, one gains a real insight into its basic constructional patterning and its relationship to other members of the animal kingdom.

SKELETON

In essence, a skeleton gives shape to an animal, the shape most characteristically seen in the animal's resting state. Skeletons, both hard and soft, use a multitalented protein called collagen as the primary scaffolding. Collagen, at a microscopic level, looks like a tri-plaited rope, technically a right-handed triple helix. These mini-fibers associate side-by-side and end-to-end to form sheets, ribbons, and cords of fascia that form an investment of pouches and pockets that envelops every bone, muscle, and organ system. Collagen is a versatile tissue that can be mineralized to form bone or hydrated to form cartilage.

A hydrostatic skeleton works by pressurizing fluids in the body via a muscular squeeze, then moving that pressurized fluid into different parts of the body, sometimes via interconnecting compartments. By changing shape in a coherent way the animal moves. Hard skeletons (both external, such as in insects, and internal, such as in humans) allow animals to get much larger and offer more powerful movement patterns as muscular force is directed via hinges and joints. Hard skeletons may complement or replace the biomechanical functions of fluid skeletons. For example, crabs periodically shed their hard external skeleton when they outgrow it, so for a period they shift to a hydrostatic-based form of movement.

SYMMETRY

Sponges are amongst the most primitive of animals. They are essentially asymmetrical. Some animals exhibit a form of radial symmetry (e.g. jellyfish), but most animals have a bilateral symmetry. Here a midline plane of symmetry creates similar left–right mirror images. Many bilaterians are asymmetrical in some features, e.g. the one large claw of the fiddler crab, and it is common for organ systems to be off center. Bilaterians tend to have an elongated anteroposterior axis that has a brain at one end and that is regionally differentiated along that axis.

Symmetry v. asymmetry is a complex topic that is discussed at all levels in science, from molecular biology to cosmology to mathematics. The contractile field (CF) model notes a key difference between the body-wall musculature and the visceral musculature – the former is bilaterally symmetrical whilst the latter is handed but asymmetrical. Our lives thus embody a profound mediation between the symmetrical and the asymmetrical.

APPENDAGES

When I studied anatomy, human limbs were presented as mere appendages, like accessories on the body-wall. You could surgically remove them and still just get by (unlike a liver or heart), and when we studied their function they were somehow divorced from the rest of the body. Manual techniques for the upper and lower limbs were taught on a different day by a different lecturer. It was a revelation to discover that limbs are in the core suite that defines body-plans – they are certainly not add-ons. Animals can have zero limbs, two limbs, four limbs, six limbs, or many limbs. We belong to the vertebrate lineage characterized by two pairs of fins/limbs where each pair has its own evolutionary and developmental history.

CLEAVAGE

Following fertilization, in all animal species known, a process called cleavage creates multicellularity. A series of divisions reduces the (often relatively enormous) volume of the fertilized egg into numerous, smaller, nucleated cells (called blastomeres).

The amount and distribution of yolk determines where cleavage can occur. At the relatively yolk-free pole of the egg (called the animal pole) the cellular divisions occur at a faster rate than at the opposite yolk-rich (vegetal) pole. Zygotes (fertilized ovums) with large yolks undergo forms of *meroblastic* cleavage, i.e. only a portion of the cytoplasm is cleaved. Examples of this pattern include most arthropods, reptiles, birds, and fishes, such as the zebrafish in Figure 1.1 (Gilbert 1997).

In zygotes with relatively little yolk, the cleavage furrow extends through the entire egg, termed *holoblastic* cleavage. Four major holoblastic cleavage patterns are observed:

1. *Radial holoblastic cleavage*: This type of cleavage is characteristic of echinoderms, as well as frogs and salamanders. The initial cleavage passes through the animal–vegetal poles creating two equal-sized daughter cells. This is termed a meridial cleavage as it passes through the two poles like a meridian on a globe. A second divisional furrow passes at right angles to this first meridial cleavage but still perpendicular to the animal–vegetal axis of the egg. The third cleavage furrow is equatorial, creating four cells above this cleavage plane in the animal half and four cells below, the vegetal half. The fourth division is again meridial, producing two tiers of eight cells each. Successive divisions alternate equatorial/meridial.

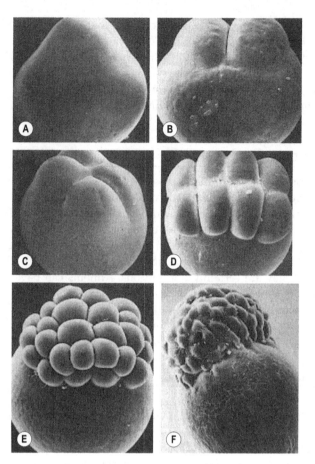

FIG 1.1 **A zebra-fish exhibiting meroblastic cleavage** Observe how the yolk-free animal pole cleaves, creating multicellularity. The yolk remains undivided. *Adapted from Gilbert 1997,* © *Gordon L. Watchmaker, formerly of Lawrence Livermore National Laboratory.*

2. *Spiral holoblastic cleavage:* Spiral cleavage is characteristic of many worms and all molluscs except cephalopods (octopus/squid, etc.). The cells do not divide in parallel or perpendicular orientations to the animal–vegetal axis of the egg. Rather, cleavage is at oblique angles, forming a 'spiral' arrangement of daughter blastomeres. In this cleavage pattern the cells touch each other more intimately than those of a radially cleaving embryo. Cleavage orientation can be to the left or right, creating left- or right-handed coiling.

3. *Bilateral holoblastic cleavage:* The most striking phenomenon in this type of cleavage is that the first cleavage plane establishes the only plane of symmetry in the embryo, separating the embryo into its future left and right sides. Bilateral holoblastic cleavage is found primarily in ascidians – the filtering and squirting invertebrates (Gilbert 1997).

4. *Rotational holoblastic cleavage:* I have introduced these arcane cleavage patterns as a backdrop for this type of cleavage, found only in mammals

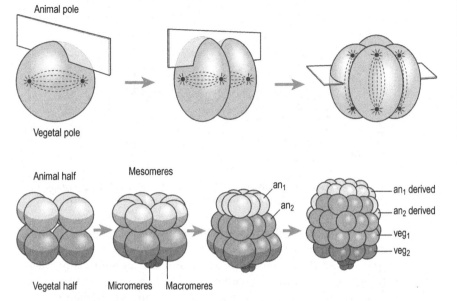

FIG 1.2 **A form of radial holoblastic cleavage in the sea urchin** *Adapted from Gilbert 1997, © Gordon L. Watchmaker, formerly of Lawrence Livermore National Laboratory.*

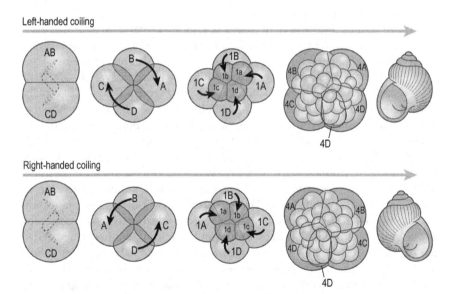

FIG 1.3 **Spiral holoblastic cleavage** Note the importance of the second cleavage cycle; the early divisions affect all subsequent development. *Adapted from Gilbert 1997, © Gordon L. Watchmaker, formerly of Lawrence Livermore National Laboratory.*

(but as is so often the case in biology, surprises are the norm as some roundworms apparently use a similar pattern). Mammalian cleavage has been difficult to study because the eggs are few, small and develop deep within the mother. Gulyas (1975), in a study based on rabbits, overcame these hurdles to discover a new cleavage pattern that is common to all

13

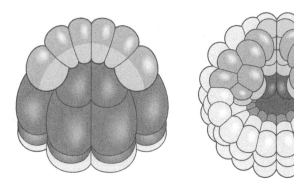

FIG 1.4 Bilateral holoblastic cleavage produces complex bodies with strict left/right symmetry.
Adapted from Gilbert 1997, © Gordon L. Watchmaker, formerly of Lawrence Livermore National Laboratory.

mammals thus observed. Termed rotational holoblastic cleavage, it is marked by the following characteristics:

(a) compared with the vast majority of the animal kingdom mammalian early cleavage rates are deliberate and slow, about 12–24 hours apart

(b) compared with most other animal embryos there is a marked asynchrony of early divisions. Usually 2–4–8, etc. cells are produced by cleavage but this rotational form frequently contains odd numbers of cells: 2–3–4–7–8 and so on. This is a much more complex developmental 'step'

(c) importantly, the pattern of cleavage is termed rotational because of a unique orientation of the cleaving force. The first cleavage is a normal meridial division; however, in the second cleavage one of the two blastomeres is cleaved meridially whilst the other cleaves equatorially.

The second cleavage is unique – it is rotational because the cleavage plane undergoes a twist of 90 degrees. If you hold a flexible plastic ruler horizontally at one end whilst twisting the far end to a perpendicular plane, the force involved by introducing this torsional dynamic to cleavage is made apparent. Blastomeres become 'torqued' together. Mammalian egg cleavage very quickly produces patterns of profound complexity that I surmise might contribute to the formation of other characteristics unique to mammals. Nipples and milk, mobile muscular lips that suck via a diaphragm, jaw joints that can move left/right as well as up/down, complexly crossed optic nerves, and a brain that is characterized by cognitive fluidity (Mithen 1996) across the corpus callosum are examples that come to mind. The contractile field model places great importance on our human ability to contra-twist the shoulders and hips which we employ to walk and throw. In principle, mammalian rotational complexity can be traced all the way back to those first cleavage cycles – the crucial first cuts of a biological cake that will become unimaginably complex.

BODY CAVITIES

An animal body has two movement imperatives – an internal imperative to move nutrients to all cells, and an external imperative to move its whole body

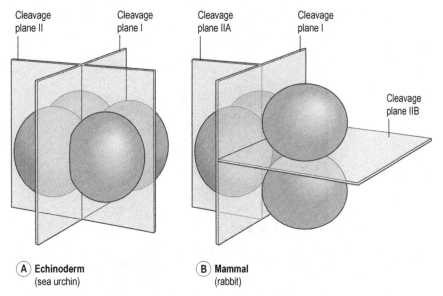

Cleavage plane II   Cleavage plane I   Cleavage plane IIA   Cleavage plane I

Cleavage plane IIB

(A) Echinoderm
(sea urchin)

(B) Mammal
(rabbit)

FIG 1.5 A comparison of early cleavage in (A) echinoderms (radial cleavage) and (B) mammals (rotational holoblastic cleavage). The second cleavage is the unusual form that twists as it cuts across the initial two cells. *Adapted from Gilbert 1997, © Gordon L. Watchmaker, formerly of Lawrence Livermore National Laboratory.*

through space for the needs of life. Often these imperatives have conflicting interests. Below is a brief introduction to the way animal body design has met this challenge via the development of body cavities.

It took life billions of years to develop the cellular biochemical pathways needed to extract food from the environment, and pass these techniques onto the next generation. Multicellularity was the next step. Cohorts of cells became bound together to form sheets of organic tissue. Some cells became specialized in dealing with the external boundary layer; this layer is termed the ectoderm in embryology. From the ectodermal layer the vertebrate central nervous system and skin came to be derived. Other cells formed an internal boundary layer that specialized in the acquisition of nutrients from the environment. This layer is called the endoderm.

Animals thus developed two thin but well-differentiated tissue layers separated by a gelatinous layer. Examples of these bilaminar animals are jellyfish, sea anemones, and comb jellies (Erwin et al 1997).

After the bilaminar body-plan came the next major innovation, an animal that produced a body built via three primary layers. During embryogenesis, a momentous event called gastrulation pours cells between the ectoderm and the endoderm, producing a new layer called mesoderm. Mesoderm is about movement. Muscle, bone, blood, and surprisingly the kidneys, are all derived from mesoderm. An example of this type of construction is the flatworm. Flatworms are flat because their trilaminar body-plan (ectoderm–mesoderm–endoderm) lacks a circulatory system so oxygen needs

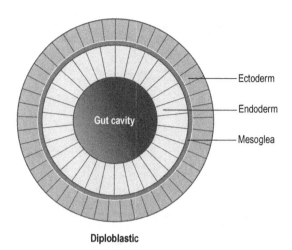

Diploblastic

FIG 1.6 Jellyfish have two distinct layers surrounding the gut cavity. *Adapted from Erwin et al 1997, reprinted by permission of American Scientist, magazine of Sigma Xi, The Scientific Research Society.*

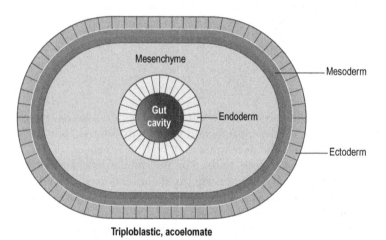

Triploblastic, acoelomate

FIG 1.7 **A three-layered flatworm** The outside layer, the ectoderm forms skin/brain. The middle layer (mesoderm) forms muscle/cartilage and bone. The endoderm forms the gut lining from mouth to anus. Flatworms have no blood system and no internal cavity – the coelom. *Adapted from Erwin et al 1997, reprinted by permission of American Scientist, magazine of Sigma Xi, The Scientific Research Society.*

to be transported to their inner tissue layers by diffusion. Small and soft-bodied, no fossil flatworms are definitely identified in the fossil record although both morphological and molecular studies concur in indicating they are amongst the earliest of animals (Erwin et al 1997).

Rounded burrows, meandering trails, and faecal pellets are traces that sponges and flatworms would be unable to leave, but 565 MYA fossil evidence of this type has been found at numerous, widely-spread, locations.

To produce such traces requires an organism that is not flat, can propel itself by generating peristaltic waves, and has a complete gut. The kinds of

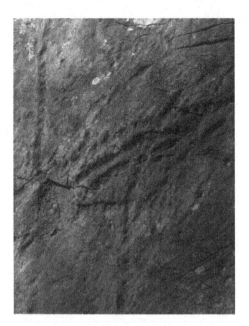

FIG 1.8 These burrows in mud are the first hard evidence of movement, about 565 MYA. This worm-like animal moved by squeezing blood up and down the length of the body. *From Erwin et al 1997, courtesy of the Smithsonian Institute.*

peristaltic locomotion that must have produced these early traces require a 'soft skeleton' of fluid-filled spaces inside a muscular sheath. A hydrostatic skeleton developed based on the compression of blood (Erwin et al 1997).

A hemocoelic (blood) space developed between the endoderm and ectoderm. Blood is a mesodermal tissue – this means it comes from the same layer of the embryo as the muscles and bones. Blood surrounded the gut tube facilitating nutrient extraction and oxygen transfer. Via large-scale blood movements the animal could change its shape. Parts of the animal might dilate whilst other parts squeeze down. All movement involves changing the shape of an organism – to move coherently an animal must be able to coherently change its shape. To burrow, muscle fibers need to be both longitudinally and horizontally placed about the body-wall. If the animal is built on a segmented plan, blood transfer then is partially partitioned. One segment may expand as others dilate, so squeezing blood about the body was an important innovation in the development of a body that could move. However, the linking of blood supply to external body movement is energetically inefficient and expensive, as the animal has to keep moving to keep a blood flow.

About 580 MYA, life was emerging from a prolonged and devastating climatic period. Out of this inferno emerged a body-plan that was to turbo-charge the evolution of animals. A triploblastic body with both a canalized hemocoel and a coelomic space emerged from the planetary chaos.

17

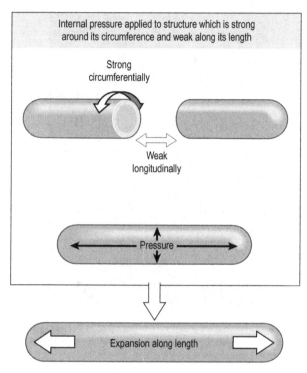

FIG 1.9 Radially squeezing a tube restores/stiffens length. From an early stage in animal design, muscles needed to align themselves both down the length of the animal and around its girth.

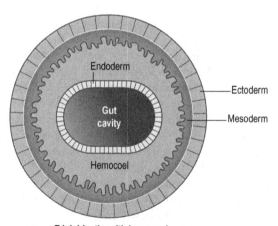

Triploblastic, with hemocoel

FIG 1.10 A triploblastic body with a hemocoel containing blood The endoderm will be the gut lining. Under the ectoderm is the muscular layer, the mesoderm. Blood is compressed between the mesodermal and endodermal layers. *Adapted from Erwin et al 1997, reprinted by permission of American Scientist, magazine of Sigma Xi, The Scientific Research Society.*

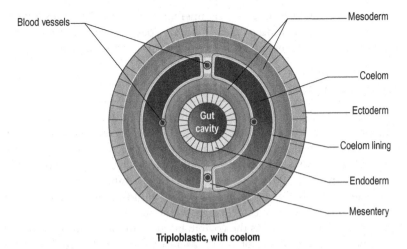

Triploblastic, with coelom

FIG 1.11 A true coelom develops within the muscular layer, the mesoderm. The mesoderm cleaves forming a fluid-filled cavity that is surrounded by muscle tissue. This created a tube within tube body-plan. The hemocoel became canalized into its own pressurized system, the cardiovascular system that keeps blood moving even when the animal is at rest. *Adapted from Erwin et al 1997, reprinted by permission of American Scientist, magazine of Sigma Xi, The Scientific Research Society.*

Blood was canalized and a pump, semi-independent of external body movement, pressurized the blood vessels. Cells throughout the body could now expect regular irrigation from blood containing oxygen and nutrients – without having to get into strange shapes to drive the blood about the body. Car engine design faced similar problems as the early engines used internal component movement to splash oil about. If the engine slowed, oil splash was also reduced – a separate oil pump sorted that issue. Animal bodies did the same but there was still a big hurdle to overcome.

If an animal had a large meal and then needed to move, the meal was moved up or down the length of the gut tube. With vigorous exertion the meal could be ejected via the mouth or anus so the gastrointestinal tract (GIT) could not develop specialist regions. A coelom was the fix.

A coelom (pronounced 'seal-um') is a fluid-filled cavity that develops within the mesodermal layer, the muscle layer of the animal. In Figure 1.11, the coelom effectively creates a body with a tube within a tube. A true coelom develops within the mesoderm whilst a pseudocoelom lies between embryonic layers. Because of a coelom the gastrointestinal system is now semi-independent of the external body-wall where all the large body-moving muscles are found. You can eat a large baguette and still run for the bus – without vomiting or defecating – thanks to this tube within tube build.

The coelomic space is found between the viscera and the external body-wall; we know its vestiges in our bodies as the peritoneal, pleural and pericardial spaces. Animals of this type now had a fundamental architecture that allowed blood to flow in well-defined pressurized vessels, had a gut tube that was directional and regionally specialized, and this internal movement largely separated from body-wall movement via a slippery coelom.

19

Vertebrates developed from this fundamental body-plan. The manipulation of fluids within the hemocoel and coelomic spaces is an essential key in understanding the earliest of movement patterns, and hence ours.

SEGMENTATION

The evolution of the coelom led to an enormous radiation of invertebrate groups of animals, but the full advantages of the coelom as a hydrostatic skeleton were not realized until the emergence of segmentation. 'A segment is a set of body parts that is present in a repeated series in an embryo or adult' (Liem et al 2001). Master genes (Hox) control segmentation; by altering the expression of these genes, bodies could be elongated or shortened by the addition or subtraction of segments. With the emergence of segmentation in some animals the coelom became divided into semi-discrete compartments, each capable of acting as reservoirs for the fluid skeleton. This enabled those animals to produce a much more efficient burrowing locomotion as exemplified by the earthworms, where different regions of the body could be in different states of dilation or contraction. This independent action of different regions of the body had further implications for the nervous system that now needed to control and coordinate the movements of different regions of the body. With the emergence of skeletons the dependence upon the coelom as a hydrostatic skeleton was reduced.

THE VERTEBRATE BODY-PLAN

The human body is a vertebrate body, a body-plan that has a long lineage. By briefly considering what defines vertebrates we gain perspective when we consider our own movement patterns.

The phylum Chordata is one of the 36(+/−) surviving body-plans to emerge from the Cambrian period. Chordates are a body-plan with the following as defining characteristics:

- A notochord (a stiffing midline rod of cartilage)
- A dorsal hollow central nervous system
- A pharynx with paired pouches and clefts in the embryo stage.

Vertebrates are chordates with vertebrae bones forming around the notochord. All vertebrates conform to a generalized pattern of anatomic structure. This is revealed by dissectional homologies and a similar pattern of embryonic development. Vertebrate development is described using four principal axes: a longitudinal (cephalic/caudal) axis, a dorso–ventral axis, and a left–right axis, with the fourth axis as a developmental time line. Vertebrates exhibit a clearly defined head with sense organs encased in capsules, external bilateral symmetry, spinal segmentation, and a coelom. Surrounding the coelom is the muscular body-wall that is continuous from the cranial base to the tail. Paired pectoral and pelvic appendages, supported by an internal skeleton and operated by contributions from the trunk musculature are also characteristic of vertebrates (Kent 1992).

The typical vertebrate body consists of four regional components: the head, the trunk, the post-anal tail, and paired pectoral and pelvic appendages. The heads of early vertebrates were solid affairs. Much evolutionary development has been directed toward opening the skull with foramina for nerves, sensory capsules, and jaw development. Concentrated in or on the head are the special sense organs that monitor the external environment and inform movement. Cephalization, based on a three-part brain, has developed to a greater degree in vertebrates than in any other body-plan.

The sensory platform leads the way, scanning the environment. Out in front is an ancient sensory system, the ability to sense chemicals in water and air. The forebrain (the telencephalon) of vertebrates is built around the olfactory sense, with the first cranial nerve (I) dedicated to this sense. Behind, and laterally, are the inner ear similar organs that act as gyroscopes helping to detect acceleration/deceleration, and correct pitch, yaw, and roll whilst swimming. The nerves for this organ are found in the back of the true brain (rhombencephalon), with information travelling via cranial nerve eight (VIII). Intermediate to the nose and ears are the eyes. Again the brain reflects this by placing the associated neural hardware behind the nose and in front of the ear area (the diencephalon), via cranial nerve two (II) which is actually not a nerve but an extrusion of the brain. Like the bridge of a ship the sensory platform acts as the interface between two worlds. The human sensory platform is about one thumb length in height as it crosses from the ear to the eye and the nose.

MUSCULOSKELETAL ANATOMY OF PRIMARY SWIMMERS

All known body-plans evolved in water. Fresh water has a density of 1000 kg/m^3 but sea water, which contains much higher concentrations of dissolved salts, has a density of 1026 kg/m^3 (Alexander 1982). Many animal tissues are denser than sea water because they contain proteins, and in some cases, inorganic crystals (bone). Much aquatic evolutionary development has therefore been devoted to buoyancy management. As vertebrate bodies are denser than water they will always tend to sink, so various strategies have emerged to counter this. Swimming upward is the simplest strategy; a horizontal forward drive coupled to uplifting hydrofoils (paired fins) is another. Like airplane wings that 'stall' at low speeds some fish need to swim constantly in order to stay up (e.g. some sharks). Many fish have buoyancy organs to help match their internal pressures to those of the water depth they prefer to live in. Buoyancy organs are the most economical means for teleosts ('modern' fish) to prevent sinking unless they swim fast or undertake large depth migrations (Alexander 1982). Fat has a lower density than water so many fish have evolved wax esters and squalene as yet another way to ensure buoyancy.

Fishes have powerful axial muscles as they use the whole body-wall in thrusting against the compressive effect of water. Fish side-bend (also called lateral flexion) to propel their bodies through the water medium. This pattern of locomotion was a very early response to driving a notochordal, bilaterally symmetrical organism through the viscosity of water. The notochord is crucial to this form of propulsion as it resists the telescoping effect of a lateral muscle mass contraction. The notochord has a spiral network of reinforcing collagen bands that may be ancestral to the morphology of the vertebrae and facet joints that tetrapods developed (Kardong 1998).

In fishes, the axial musculature arises directly from the embryonic segments that form on either side of the notochord from the post-cranial region to the tail. In the adult these blocks of muscle retain their segmentation and are called myomeres. Caudally-angled connective tissue sheets, the myosepta, separate myomeres. They are internally continuous with the vertebral column. The myomeres are divided into dorsal (epaxial), and ventral (hypaxial) muscle masses by a fibrous sheet, the horizontal skeletogenous septum.

Each spinal nerve that supplies a myomere bifurcates. The dorsal ramus supplies the epaxial division, and the ventral ramus supplies the hypaxial division. Our spines retain this pattern of innervation.

With the skin removed, the myosepta of fish appear as zigzag blocks that extend into the body-wall with caudally-orientated muscular cones that look like a stack of tall caps (Kent 1992). Cones extend tendons from the muscular apex of the body-wall to the tail vertebrae, thus focusing multisegmental power for caudally-derived propulsion.

A thin sheet of oblique muscle fibers lies superficial to the main hypaxial mass in most fish. Obliquely orientated muscle allows a fish to lateral bend and twist, as seen when a fish is landed. Another muscle band is commonly present that parallels the ventral midline (linea alba), the rectus abdominus. Terrestrial vertebrates will build on these small muscles (Wake 1979).

APPENDICULAR MUSCULATURE

The gills interrupt the segmentation of the hypaxial muscles of fishes, and where the pectoral and pelvic girdles are embedded in the body-wall. The appendicular muscles of fishes are uncomplicated, exhibit little variety and perform a restricted function, that of stability/guidance in a fluid medium.

Streamlining is a biological imperative as speed increases. Shapes that evolved within water and were streamlined soon encountered the problem of three-dimensional stability. Any streamlined body travelling at speed has a tendency to tip and deviate from its line of travel, rotating about its center of mass. It may swing from side to side (yaw), rock about its long axis (roll), or may tip upward or downward (pitch). Appropriately positioned stabilizing fins counter these directional deviations (Kardong 1998).

The body-wall of the primitive fish carries projecting spines, lobes, or processes. Unlike these projections, fins are membranous or webbed processes internally strengthened by radiating, thin dermal fin rays. Fins occur singly, except for the pectoral and pelvic bilaterally symmetrical fins, the phylogenic (the evolution of development through a succession of forms) source of tetrapod limbs. The origin of paired fins is one of the more puzzling questions in the study of phylogeny. As they are part of the definition of the vertebrate body-plan they must be ancient and deeply conserved. *At the Water's Edge* by Carl Zimmer (1999) is a fascinating read about how, when, and where fins morphed into limbs.

Fin musculature is derived from embryonic myomeres (the migrating precursor of muscle) near the base of each fin fold. A fin fold is a pinching of the ventro/lateral body-wall. The precursor muscle cells invade fin buds to establish dorsal and ventral muscle masses called moieties (halves). Dorsal muscle moieties form extensors (or abductors, or elevators, or external rotators – all these terms are used); ventral moieties form the flexors (adductors, depressors, internal rotators). Complexity is generated when the fin bud twists so that fluid dynamics across the fin can be exquisitely controlled.

The next step in this story is to briefly look at the embryogenesis of the key anatomical structures that generate our movement. Then we are in a position to begin the task of constructing a model of mammalian movement that attempts to be congruent with these disciplines.

REFERENCES

Alexander R 1982 Locomotion of animals. Blackie, Glasgow

Arthur W 1997 The origin of animal body plans. Cambridge University Press, Cambridge

Erwin D, Valentine J, Jablonski D 1997 The origin of animal body plans. American Scientist 85:126–137

Gilbert S 1997 Developmental biology, 5th edn. Sinauer Associates Inc, Sunderland

Gulyas B 1975 A reexamination of the cleavage patterns in eutherian mammalian eggs: rotation of the blastomere pairs during second cleavage in the rabbit. Journal of Experimental Zoology 193:235–248

Hamilton G 2005 Looking for LUCA – the mother of all life. New Scientist 2515:26

Hamilton G 2008 Viruses: the unsung heroes of evolution. New Scientist 2671:38–41

Kardong K 1998 Vertebrates: comparative anatomy, function, evolution, 2nd edn. WCB/McGraw-Hill, Boston

Kent G 1992 Comparative anatomy, 7th edn. Mosby, St Louis

Liem K, Bemis W, Walker W, Grande L 2001 Functional anatomy of the vertebrates. An evolutionary perspective, 3rd edn. Harcourt College Publishers, Fort Worth

McMenamin M, McMenamin D 1990 The emergence of animals. Columbia University Press, New York

Mithen S 1996 The prehistory of the mind. Thames and Hudson, London

Raff R 1996 The shape of life. University of Chicago Press, Chicago

Wake M 1979 Hyman's comparative vertebrate anatomy, 3rd edn. University of Chicago Press, Chicago

Zimmer C 1999 At the water's edge: fish with fingers, whales with legs, and how life came ashore but then went back to the sea. Touchstone, New York

Embryological morphogenesis

2

Embryology is an exercise in time reversal. By returning to the initial stages of our development we gain perspective, insight, and humility in the presence of awesome morphogenesis.

'A wriggle in deep time' took a phylogenic look – the evolution of development through a succession of forms – at the vertebrate body plan. This chapter takes an ontogenic perspective – which is the study of an individual organism's development from conception to maturity. My remit here is to briefly introduce prenatal life, dwelling principally on the external shape and form of the embryo – its morphology.

Embryology is hidden and arcane. It has a specialized language that describes structures and processes that are, particularly in the first few weeks, in a state of awe-inspiring flux. The extraordinary three-dimensional interplay of the viscera, muscles, and nerves requires of the reader a spatial gymnastic to comprehend. But the subject is worth the effort as each one of us has experienced this process personally. As Aristotle noted, 'One who sees things from the beginning will have the finest view of them.'

Let us look at the size and time frame. A fertilized ovum is about half the size of a full stop on this page and weighs 15 ten millionths of a gram (Wendell & Williams 1984). The following 8 post-fertilization weeks are called the embryonic period. During this time the single fertilized ovum repeatedly cleaves (via that dynamic called rotational holoblastic cleavage) to produce a ball of cells that then compact and waft down the fallopian tube, implanting

25

DOI: 10.1016/B978-0-7020-3109-0.00007-9

the now morula-like ball of cells in the uterine lining. During the next 7 weeks the embryo generates an astounding internal complexity. It has been estimated that over 90% of all the named structures of the adult body are present at 8 weeks, when the embryo is less than half the length of your thumb (O'Rahilly & Müller 1996).

The fetal period covers weeks 8–30: growth and remodelling of structures laid down earlier prepares the fetus for birth, by then weighing about 3.4 kg, a 2.3 thousand millions weight increase from fertilization. Embryology texts are usually 200–400 pages long so here I will dwell on only those aspects of this arcane subject that are pertinent to the CF model of movement. Please use the reference list to follow up on this introduction, and accept the necessary simplifications inherent in a one-chapter introduction to this fascinating subject. I will present the following introduction to embryology in part as a story directed to your imagination.

You are a large, round fertilized cell, a unique fusion of your paternal and maternal genetic adventures. A huge internal force cleaves you from the north pole to the south pole, thus producing two cells. Again, you cleave – one cell is split along the equator; the cleaving force twists 90 degrees and continues cutting the second cell longitudinally, cleaving slowly and deliberately. Now you are four human cells, complexly rotationally bonded together. Do mammals have special access to rotational biodynamics because of this cleavage pattern? The fallopian tubes gently wave and float your tumbling cleaving cell mass toward the uterus.

COMPACTION

Mammals cleave via rotational holoblastic cleavage. They then experience a 'compaction event' that huddles the tiny morula of cells tightly together – responsibilities are established that last a lifetime.

Following another couple of cleavage cycles, something amazing suddenly happens to you. Think shrink-wrap! Termed the 'compaction' event, it is as unique and important to mammals as rotational holoblastic cleavage. Imagine yourself as a group of about 8–16 cells, all close friends but all with a little fluid between you that allows slip and jostle as you trade. Each of these initial cells is considered to be totipotent, i.e. each is capable of forming any body part. These initial few cells are not identical but they do have a large range of competencies. Compaction changes that; the rotational bonds between cells must reach a tipping point that suddenly torques down, creating a compacted, tightly bonded morula (mulberry-like) of cells. Now you are hugging your friends in tight embrace. Intercellular communication moves from 'dial-up' to 'high-speed broadband'. During compaction it is decided which of these few cells will form the embryo body, and which will form the packaging around the embryo.

A day or two later the morula has completed a long journey without much sustenance. You feel an imperative to embed yourself in a rich uterine lining, which you must do during your second week. Landing on the uterine lining, with what will eventually be your back, causes a wholesale rearrangement of your inner cells.

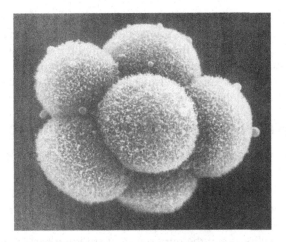

FIG 2.1   Scanning electron micrograph of a mouse embryo that is uncompacted *From Bloom 1989, with permission.*

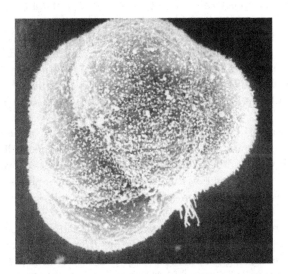

FIG 2.2   Compacted mouse embryo The morula appears to have been shrink-wrapped. The microvilla are found now only on the external surface. *From Bloom 1989, with permission.*

BILAMINAR EMBRYONIC DISC

During days 12–17 the embryonic cells proliferate and migrate via a form of involution. The longitudinal axis is established, giving the embryo bilateral symmetry.

Two distinct cell layers emerge, the epiblast and the hypoblast, that together are known as the embryonic disc. These two layers complexly transform with the epiblast contributing the lion's share of what will be the embryo proper. The hypoblast goes on to form the placenta and membranes around the embryo (to be later discarded as the afterbirth). Your 'back' at this stage is the epiblast, which develops a fluid cushion behind it (called the amniotic cavity, which will eventually surround you); your 'front' sports a fluid cavity that will be your small yolk-sac. Surrounding the embryonic disc is a much larger fluid sac called the blastocystic cavity. You do not have much fuel on board so you bury yourself deeper into the fluid-rich warmth of the uterus whilst sending rather insistent emissaries that arrange for a hook-up to your mother's uterine glands and circulation. You were expected. The second week establishes a relationship that is vital to all that follows, for both you and your mother.

GASTRULATION AND THE PRIMITIVE STREAK/NODE/PIT

Gastrulation initiates the formation of a trilaminar disc, the notochord, and the onset of organogenesis.

Lewis Wolpert (1986) famously contends 'It is not birth, marriage, or death, but gastrulation, which is truly the most important time in your life.' Wolpert (1991, p. 12) goes on to say 'Excessive perhaps, but the occasion was the attempt to convince the clinician of the importance of studying early development.'

Gastrulation occurs in the development of all animals. As in cleavage, the details of gastrulation vary in pattern across and even within phyla. At 2 weeks, the embryo is termed diploblastic as it consists of two flat layers of cells, the epiblast and the hypoblast. The bilaminar disc is converted to a tri-laminar disc via the morphing, called gastrulation. The new layer is called mesoderm, termed an intermediate germ layer as it is spread between the outside layer and the new inside layer. All trilaminar animal groups use the vast, migratory cellular dynamics initiated during gastrulation to bring cells from the outside layer of the embryo to the interior. A form of involution takes place.

Imagine yourself now at that stage in your life. You are entering your third week post conception. You have already established a life-long rela-tionship with your mother. You are shaped like a flattened pear, have two layers, and are surrounded by fluid contained by delicate life-support mem-branes. Your sense of direction is hazy. Head and tail, left and right have little meaning to you.

Gastrulation gives a left/right laterality by initiating a process that will cleave your epiblastic 'back' in the midline from the caudal toward the cephalic region. During gastrulation, huge numbers of cells are on the move – the whole embryo is heaving, involuting, invaginating in and through itself. The cellular choreography is astoundingly three-dimensionally complex – even a slight aberration will crash the nascent biological system. The Indian tradition talks of 'the kundalini', a powerful coiled energy moving from caudal to rostral that they associate with spiritual illumination. If you could re-experience even a small percentage of the feeling involved in the gastrula-tion event, your life subsequently would be altered by that physiological tsunami. Wisely, the Indian seers also warn of a great danger if this re-arousal of the serpent power goes awry.

The cleaving running up your middle dorsal surface is like a long fault line into which your epiblastic cells are irresistibly drawn by strong currents – Niagara Falls springs to mind. The cleavage is called the 'primitive streak' and at its cephalic end, it is a midline rounded structure, the 'primitive node' that surrounds the 'primitive pit' (embryology's metaphoric equivalent of a cosmic black hole).

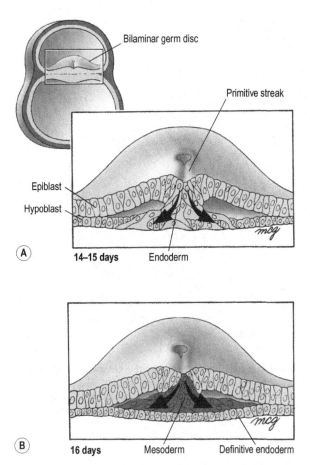

Bilaminar germ disc

Primitive streak

Epiblast

Hypoblast

(A) **14–15 days** Endoderm

(B) **16 days** Mesoderm Definitive endoderm

FIG 2.3 The bilaminar disc invaginates (the outside becomes the inside) and in so doing, creates the middle germ layer, the mesoderm. *Adapted from Schoenwolf et al 2008.*

As thousands of cells pour over the lip of the primitive streak they undergo profound, lasting metamorphosis. Cells from the epiblast are transformed into the definitive trilaminar embryo. Epiblastic cells dislodge the hypoblast and form what is now called the definitive endoderm. Endoderm, the deepest of the three germ layers, forms the cells that line your gut tube from mouth to anus. Between the newly forming endoderm and the epiblast a new cell layer is created by the in-pouring epiblastic cells, the mesoderm, forming in time, muscle, bone, blood, and the genito-urinary system. The outside germ layer, the epiblast, is now transformed into a layer called the ectoderm, from which the skin and nervous system are derived. Thus, three definitive germ layers are now present: the endoderm, the mesoderm, and the ectoderm.

One of the defining characteristics of vertebrates is an embryonic structure called the notochord. All vertebrates have a notochord, if only at this stage of their development. It arises as a cephalic continuation of the primitive pit; in Figure 2.4 it will project forward from the horseshoe-shaped primitive pit. Within the softly structured body of the embryo the notochord is a tough midline rod of cartilage that forms during days 16–31, a rod of spirally bound,

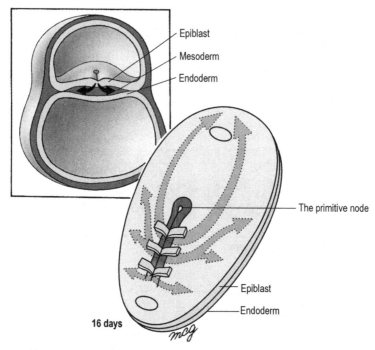

Epiblast

Mesoderm

Endoderm

The primitive node

Epiblast

Endoderm

16 days

FIG 2.4 Where epiblastic cells fall into the primitive streak and node determines the trajectory of their subsequent migration The oval depicted above the primitive node is the oral membrane – it is a tight pinching of the epiblast and hypoblast – it will be the future mouth region. Likewise, the caudal oval will be the cloacal region (anus).
Adapted from Schoenwolf et al 2008.

fluid-engorged cells that resists being shortened. Dorsal to the notochord will lie the central nervous system; ventral to the notochord will be the gut tube and the heart tubes. Both the gut tube and spinal cord require a notochord for correct development, i.e. the notochord is an inductive agent. Induction is an important concept in embryology that speaks of early affinities and influences across germ layers (Larsen 1993). One group of embryonic cells signals to another group of cells so that the second group is initiated to further develop via a new permission or instruction. For example, the notochord induces mesoderm to materialize.

FOLDING

The process known as folding creates the shape of the embryo, both external and internal. A knowledge of embryonic folding explains how many muscles come to migrate long distances from their site of origin.

Now the embryo 'folds'. The illustration in Figure 2.6 maps out the parts of the ovoid germ disc that will be assigned to different body parts. Folding creates a three-dimensional shape from the flattened trilaminar germ disc. At this stage, the fourth week, the notochord and the newly created mesoderm that will form the segmented vertebrae and muscles act as a stiffened

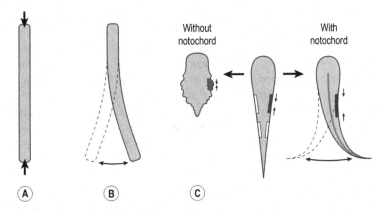

FIG 2.5 All vertebrates have a notochord for good reason Without a notochord the locomotion system that is based on side-bending could not have evolved, as muscle contraction one side of the body would have shortened, telescope-like, that side. *Adapted from Kardong 1998, with permission.*

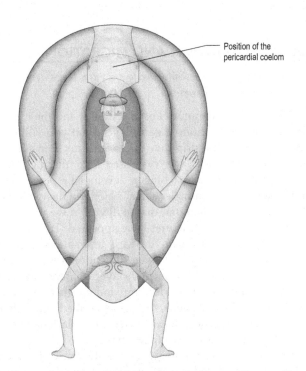

Position of the pericardial coelom

FIG 2.6 A bilaminar disc before the folding event, looking at this stage like a flattened pear The pinched oval regions mark the site of the future mouth and anal region. Note how the cardiogenic region at this stage is above the future brain on the bilaminar disc. The lower abdominal region is below the anal region. *Adapted from Standring 2008.*

longitudinal brace. Folding occurs primarily in the thin flexible rim of the embryonic disc. The left and right disc margins fold ventrally, called lateral flexion. Concurrently, the top and bottom of the disc fold ventrally, called longitudinal flexion. Folding drags the future brain, organs, and pioneer muscle cells with it.

31

Lateral folding drags the precursors of muscle and bone from the back of the embryonic body out to the sides and then to the ventral midline. Concurrently, at the top of the embryonic disc the cells that will contribute to the future heart are gathered. With longitudinal folding, your future 'heart' is dragged from this position ventrally toward what will be the anterior chest. Quite literally, you are led by the heart's migration into the chest wall – pushed there by the brain's massive growth. Under the heart, and attached to it, is the central area of the diaphragm (at this stage called the septum transversum). As it descends to the thorax, it excavates muscle tissue from the interior chest wall to form part of its muscular attachments to the ribs and lumbar vertebrae.

The caudal region is also pulled ventrally. Tissue that was on the sacrococcygeal region of the body is drawn to the ventral region where it contributes to the formation of the pelvic floor, the genitalia, and the lower abdominal wall. Folding from the cephalic region meets folding from the caudal region just below the navel. Traditional Chinese Medicine (TCM) gives this region of the body great importance, the Dantian or the field of elixir.

MESODERMAL FORMATION AND MIGRATION

Mesoderm, the middle of the three embryonic layers, forms bones, tendons, muscles, blood, and kidneys. Mesoderm moves us.

The early bilaminar disc is composed of the epiblast and the hypoblast. Only the epiblast will form the definitive germ layers that you will emerge from. Epiblastic cells pour into the primitive streak and pit, transform into endoderm, ectoderm, and the new layer discussed here, the mesoderm. With a mesodermal layer, animals became bigger, developed a powerful body musculature, and larger organs. Animals with a mesoderm developed real vigour.

Figure 2.7A illustrates a trilaminar disc at day 18. A week later the embryo has folded and many named structures have appeared. The outside layer, the ectoderm, has morphed into the skin, the early brain and spinal cord, and all the nerves that emanate. The inner layer, the endoderm, has started on its journey to form the gut tube, the absorptive layer from mouth to anus. Mesoderm is pulled ventrally via lateral folding, and concurrently, mesoderm at the top and bottom of the embryonic disc is also pulled ventrally (longitudinal folding). Thus the embryonic disc, which is like a flattened pear, becomes, with folding, a three-dimensional tadpole shape.

Three regions of mesoderm emerge. Along the back of the embryo is a longitudinally semi-segmented mass of mesoderm called the somites that will form the vertebral column, and the muscles that will power that column (the complex erector spinae group).

Migrating further laterally, another column of mesoderm forms, the intermediate mesoderm. This interesting column of mesoderm pulls away and drops deeper into the embryo to form bilateral urogenital ridges from which the kidneys and gonads will emerge. These urogenital ridges in early embryogenesis extend all the way up the length of the anterior spine to the lower neck somites. Their development is closely related to the concurrent development of the coelom. I will come back to the development of the kidneys later

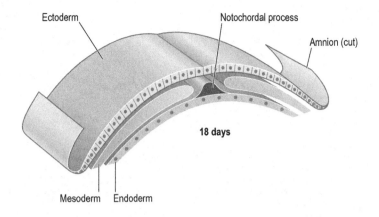

Ectoderm

Notochordal process

Amnion (cut)

18 days

Mesoderm   Endoderm

(A)

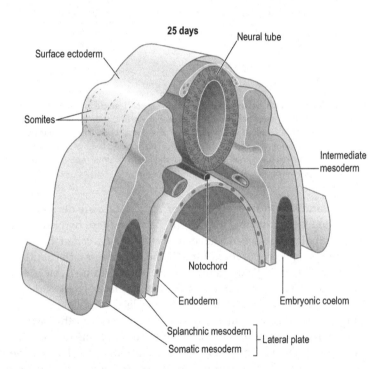

25 days

Neural tube

Surface ectoderm

Somites

Intermediate mesoderm

Notochord

Endoderm

Embryonic coelom

Splanchnic mesoderm ⎤
                    ⎦ Lateral plate
Somatic mesoderm

(B)

FIG 2.7 **Lateral folding** Mesoderm is drawn ventro-laterally to form three discernable regions: somatic, intermediate, and lateral plate. The lateral plate comprises two layers. The outside layer of the lateral plate (the somatic) forms the body-wall muscles and limbs, the inside layer (the splanchnic) forming the muscular layer of the gut tube and most of the cardiovascular muscle. The coelom is the cavity between the two contractile layers. *Adapted from Fitzgerald & Fitzgerald 1978.*

in the text as the contractile field model has a fluid field (F-F) that intermediates between the dorsal body and the ventral body.

The mesoderm lateral to the intermediate mesoderm is called the lateral plate. The lateral plate splits into two leaves. Your body wall (ribs, torso muscles, limbs) is formed by the outer leaf called the somatic mesoderm. The

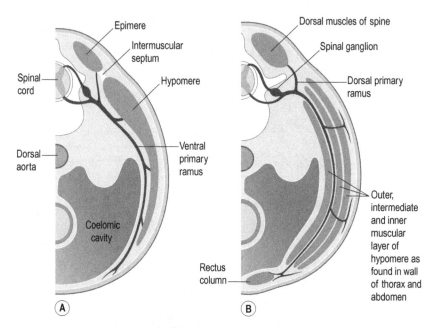

FIG 2.8 Mesodermal tissue splitting into discrete muscle masses As the intermediate mesoderm detaches and drops inward to form the urogenital organs, a partial septum is created between the muscle over the dorsal body and the outside leaf of the lateral plate, the somatic mesoderm. This somatic layer of the lateral plate splits into a trilaminar body-wall and a rectus abdominis column. *Adapted from Sandler 1990, with kind permission of Lippincott, Williams and Wilkins. http://lww.com.*

muscles and supportive structures of your viscera are derived from the inner leaf, called the splanchnic mesoderm. Between these two leaves of contractile mesodermal tissue a fluid-filled cavity develops called the coelom, which from the perspective of the contractile field model is a particularly important structure. Figure 2.7B shows the somites, the yet-to-be-detached intermediate mesoderm, and the two layers of the lateral plate.

Figure 2.8 shows the somatic (the outer leaf) mesoderm being pulled ventrally. A split develops in the muscle tissue between the back muscles and the lateral plate mesoderm. The adult position of this mesodermal split is in the region of the rib angles on your dorsal body wall. The muscle that encircles the embryo lateral to this line of demarcation (the somatic mesoderm) splits into three layers. All mammals have a trilaminar body wall, three distinct layers of muscle that form the deep, intermediate, and superficial layers of the chest and abdominal wall. When the left and right lateral folding of the embryo approach the ventral midline, another muscle split is seen, marked by an abrupt muscle fiber direction change as the rectus abdominis column of muscle appears.

THE COELOM

A fluid-filled cavity, the coelom, semi-isolates visceral organ movement from body-wall and limb movement. Pericarditis, pleurisy, and peritonitis will stop an Olympic athlete from moving.

When I was first introduced to embryology the coelom was deemed by me to be a complex bit of arcane plumbing and of little clinical use to a manual therapist, so I turned those pages. I was wrong. As noted in Chapter 1, the coelom is a key characteristic in the origins and definition of a body plan. It is, in essence, a fluid-filled space or cavity that allows the viscera to be semi-independent of the body-wall. There are a number of ways of constructing a coelom, as comparative evolutionary anatomy has discovered. Primitive body-plans do not have a coelom hence they are called acoelomate. Some body-plans are built with a coelom that fits between the endoderm and mesoderm germ layers: this type is called a pseudocoelom. A split within the mesodermal layer forms a definitive coelom. Moving the coelom from underneath to within mesoderm has profound implications for animal movement.

Imagine holding a small bag of gel in your open hand. You can move your hand and thus move the gel bag but with little control of either the bag or its contents. If you place your other hand on top of that gel bag, not only can you now move the gel bag horizontally but it can now be moved in many planes, even upside down, but also you can squeeze the gel bag and manipulate its gel content. The coelom is the gel bag with one hand being represented by the muscle of the body wall, the other hand represented by the muscular tissue of the viscera. Placing the coelom within the mesoderm allowed muscle to manipulate it.

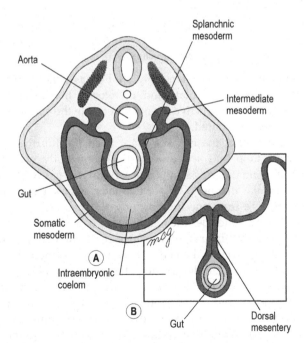

FIG 2.9 Coelom formation Mesoderm migrates laterally and ventrally forming somites, intermediate mesoderm (that will drop away to form the urogenital system), and lateral plate mesoderm that splits into two leaves that surround the coelom. The external leaf, the somatic mesoderm, forms the external trilaminar body-wall. The internal leaf, the splanchnic mesoderm, forms the gut musculature and aspects of the cardiovascular system. *Adapted from Schoenwolf et al 2008.*

In the earliest stages of embryology during the third week, a fluid-filled space that is called the extra-embryonic coelom surrounds the embryo. Later that week, as the embryo undergoes extraordinary morphogenesis, coelomic spaces within the body of the embryo coalesce to form small vesicles that then become horseshoe-like in shape to form a continuous cavity that surrounds the heart and most of the early gut tube. At this stage the two ends of the horseshoe-shaped coelom open out of the embryo body to exchange fluids with the extra-embryonic coelom. There is a commonality of the fluids of the body at this stage in embryogenesis that I will refer to when I introduce a fluid field (F-F) that is associated with the kidneys. With further development the intra-embryonic coelom is cut off from the extra-embryonic coelom and then forms discrete compartments. In the adult we know the remnants of the intra-embryonic coelom as three compartments, which are the:

- Pericardial coelom that lies between the pericardial sac and the heart (enabling the heart to pulsate at 80 beats per minute without pulsing your whole body to its beat)
- Pleural coelom that lies between the internal thoracic wall and the external surface of the lungs
- Peritoneal coelom that lies between the deep layer of the muscular abdominal wall and the abdominal viscera.

LIMB BUDS

Limbs emerge from the body-wall of the embryo as small buds that quickly become large muscular structures. Knowing how, when, and where they develop aids understanding and hence treatment of these complex structures.

Limb development has been extensively studied as it is relatively easy to remove blocks of tissue and rotate and/or relocate that block to see what happens. In this way, the inductive events that create the cardinal axes of the limb bud have been elucidated.

Human limb morphogenesis takes place from the fourth to the eighth week. The upper limb bud appears on the lateral body wall as a small, ventro/laterally orientated ridge, opposite cervicals C5 to C8. The lower limb bud arises in a similar manner a day or two later, opposite lumbar L3 to L5.

Limb buds emerge from specific portions of a transitory, intermediately placed ring that briefly encircles the whole embryo, the enigmatic ectodermal ring (also called the Wolffian ridge). During day 22, three longitudinal bands can be seen on the surface of the embryo: somatic, intermediate, and lateral plate. The somatic band straddles the dorsal midline and includes the repeating blocks of tissue (somites) that will form much of the spinal complex. Lateral plate mesoderm will, in due course, form the body wall and the deep leaf will contribute to the muscles of the viscera. The intermediate band, which overlies nephrogenic tissue (kidneys and gonads) and the coelom, is the site of the ectodermal ring. By day 24 the ridge is complete rostrally and by day 26 the ridge is completed caudally. Limb buds are emergent from the ectodermal ring on day 28. By day 37 the ectodermal ring has fully regressed. Here is a transitory, intermediate structure that is a link between the rostral/caudal, the left/right and the ventro/dorsal poles of the embryo.

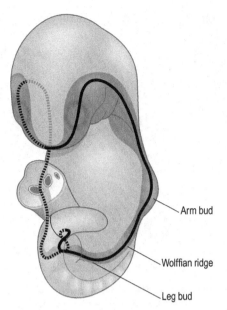

Arm bud

Wolffian ridge

Leg bud

FIG 2.10 Day 28 The ectodermal (Wolffian) ring. The ring covers the primordia of the nose, eyes, ears, vagus nerve, upper limb bud, nipple, lower limb bud, and genital tip. The ring is intermediate to the dorsal somites and the ventral visceral organs. Both the dorsal body and the ventral body contribute to the ridge of the ectodermal ring. It overlies the early stages of kidney development and the coelom before it is compartmentalized. *From Carlson 2009, based on studies by O'Rahilly & Gardner 1975.*

The ectodermal ring is also called the Wolffian ridge, the source of some historical confusion (Stephens 1982). In 1759, Casper F. Wolff noted this ridge in chick embryos but he did not name it, rather William Hiss attributed the ridge to him in a paper dated 1868. Wolff has been remembered for his apparently beautiful descriptions of the mesonephros, a transitory aspect of kidney development that will be revisited later in the text. The importance of the ectodermal ring was lost for many years, overshadowed by that description of the 'Wolffian duct.' O'Rahilly and Müller (1985) re-described the ring in great detail.

Posterior to the ring lie the somites, and anterior to the ring lie the large visceral swellings, hence the ring's designation as 'intermediate.' All of the body parts touched by the Wolffian ridge are of huge biological value and all come to be massively represented on the sensory cerebral cortex. This remarkable intermediate morphological structure links the precursor tissues of the nose, eyes, and ears with the vagus nerve, the upper limbs, the nipples, the lower limbs, and genital tip into one cohesive interconnectedness at a critical stage in embryology.

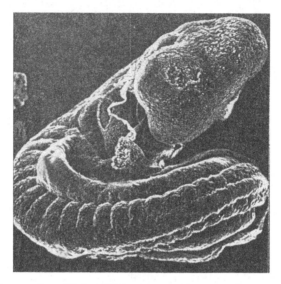

FIG 2.11 **Embryo at about 28 days** The head is built around a large fore and mid brain. No face is discernable. The cut membranes mark the removal of the heart and placenta. Somites on the dorsal body will become the spine and attendant muscles. Intermediate to the organs and somite is the Wolffian ridge from which the limb buds will emerge. To see the Wolffian ridge (or ectodermal ring) so clearly is very rare. The early swelling of the upper limb bud is visible. *Reproduced courtesy of Robert O. Kelley.*

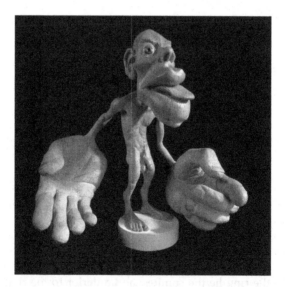

FIG 2.12 **A sensory homunculus that represents how much neural tissue is devoted to different parts of your body** Your mouth, nose, eyes, ears, hands, the nipple line, the feet, and genital tip – everything your brain is interested in was linked morphologically by the Wolffian ridge. © *The Natural History Museum, London, reproduced with permission.*

A number of observations may be made about the Wolffian ridge:

1. The ridge is probably homologous to the fin fold from which the fins of fish emerge. Fins developed in response to the evolutionary demands of fluid dynamics. Pitch, yaw, and roll are corrected for by the fins and the fin-rays. Fins are exquisitely positioned on the body wall of a fish to control and direct its drive in water. Likewise, our limbs are positioned on the body wall so that they may optimally control and (in a terrestrial environment) empower whole organism movement.

2. Vertebrate developmental biology is embedded in four dimensions: head/tail, front/back, left/right – and a time line. The timing of events in embryology is critical. Sometimes a few minutes can make a significant difference to development. Complex inductive signalling must course through the ridge as precisely timed cascades. Although little is known of the mechanisms (Carlson 1994) the Wolffian ridge must be involved with the co-development of modules (like eyes and limbs) that need tightly integrated 'inductive' cascades to form a viable whole. The Wolffian ridge must be infused with coursing inductive nectars that initiate developmental cascades.

3. The Wolffian ridge communicates with, and draws from, both the somatic and visceral domains of the embryonic body-wall. Somatic and visceral meet, like the two land masses that collided to push up the Himalayan mountain range. Underlying embryonic structures are involved in the formation of the ridge, specifically the coelom and kidney precursor tissues that, at this stage, extend up to the 'neck' region. Later in the text I will expand on this relationship between the coelom and the kidneys to propose a fluid field. In essence, all animal movement is derived from the coherent manipulation of bodily fluids. Change the volume or salinity of fluids and all physiology changes.

4. The 'phylotypic stage' of development is a brief period when all vertebrates express their core common characteristics – notochord, pharyngeal arches, fin/limb buds, bilateral symmetry, etc. (Raff 1996). Fish, crocodiles, lemurs, bats and humans, all look their most morpho-logically similar at this embryological stage. A deeply embedded, shared history is evident during this brief period in development when the fin/limbs are just emerging from the body wall.

    a. Modules of development (such as eyes and limbs) are at their most evolutionary conserved but developmentally co-dependant stage.

    b. Prior to the phylotypic stage the nascent embryo is biologically malleable (Raff 1996). Cells are more transmutable, and whole stages of development may be modified yet still yield a viable embryo. For example, some species of frogs miss the whole tadpole stage yet still emerge as competent frogs.

    c. Post phylotypic stage the embryo is now characterized by modules of development that are semi-autonomous. A teratogenic drug like thalidomide may knock out a whole developmental process, a module, in this case the limbs, but leave the rest of the baby intact.

    d. The phylotypic stage is characterized by global interaction between widely separated modules of development. It appears plausible to suggest the transient Wolffian ridge is the phylotypic stage as the ridge is emergent at the right time and it is briefly global in its embryological reach.

5. Everything that the Wolffian ridge touches comes to be massively represented on the sensory cortex of the brain. Nose, eyes, ears, vagus nerve, hands, nipples, feet, and genitals – all are touched by this transient emergence.

6. A student at the British School of Osteopathy in London, Marcia Hugal, approached me after a class to suggest the Wolffian ridge could be twisted in such a way that it forms a Möbius loop, something I had never heard of. Marcia demonstrated how to form a Möbius loop and went on to make a model with little limb buds to demonstrate the idea.

The Möbius loop

August Ferdinand Möbius was a prolific 19th-century German mathematician and astronomer who explored, amongst many things, the math involved in twisting strips of paper. This profound party trick works best if you actually do it, so I suggest you cut three or four strips of paper that are about 3 cm wide and 30 cm long, and have pencils, glue, and scissors at hand.

Firstly, just fold a paper strip so that a simple circular loop is formed. Notice that the loop has a clearly separated inside and outside surface, and two distinct edges. Information can be imprinted on both sides, but the inside is forever distinct from the outside. Now fold the paper strip with a twist of 180 degrees, and glue the two ends together, as in Figure 2.13.

The two surfaces become one continuous loop, now with only one edge. Run a pencil line down the middle of the loop and you will return to the start. The notion of inside and outside is lost. Encoded information can be processed as a continuum rather than as two discrete packages and, I hypothesize, information has a much higher transfer speed through the loop. Does molecular information feel the same rush we do when we ride a twisting roller-coaster?

I suggest the Wolffian ridge is not only a Möbius loop but a longitudinally divided loop. Why, and what does this mean? The clue is in the limb buds. Each limb consists of a core of mesoderm covered by an ectodermal cap called the apical ectodermal ridge (AER), which is a beautiful linear ridge cresting the bud (see Fig. 2.15). It is a 'strict' demarcation of the ventral/dorsal domains of the limb bud.

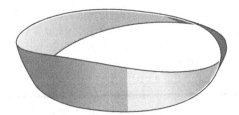

FIG 2.13 **A Möbius loop – enigmatic beauty** A simple loop had the inside shaded light gray, the outside darker gray. A 180-degree twist creates a Möbius loop that now has one continuous surface and one continuous edge. © *David Benbennick, reproduced with permission.*

The formation of the limb bud needs inducing agents from both the ventral body and the ectoderm. The ectoderm competent to form a limb bud appears to reside solely at the border between the dorsal and ventral surfaces of the embryo (Gilbert 1997). The AER is derived from the Wolffian ridge and it is evidently a dorso/ventro summation of that structure, so this suggests to me a midline splitting is possible, in principle, throughout the Wolffian ridge.

Following this idea, take another paper strip and fold it into a Möbius loop. With a pencil, run a line along the midline width of the loop. Then cut the Möbius loop down the midline – interestingly you end up with not two loops but one longer loop with another twist added.

Instead of one twist to create a Möbius loop, you can twist the paper twice (360 degrees), or you can cut the loop into thirds, or you can draw oblique lines on each side of the paper before the loop is formed – many variants on a theme that all produce unexpected outcomes. I am convinced Möbius loop dynamics are part of the morphogenic repertoire used during early cellular migration. From the onset, the embryo is a viable whole that quickly generates hundreds of named structures, but first and foremost it is a viable whole. Marcia opened my eyes to a new form of pattern generation.

Let us leave speculation on the Möbius loop and the ectodermal ring and move on with limb bud development. I will describe the upper limb first. As it emerges from the Wolffian ridge it is orientated laterally and slightly ventrally. The paddle shapes that will be the hands soon become manifest and the 'hands' then migrate to point toward the front by flexing at the new elbows, that now face laterally. Note that at this stage of embryogenesis the heart is a massive pulsating organ, pumping at 120–160 beats per minute. The growth of the heart, unrestrained by ribs, is so pronounced, it comes to nearly touch the brain that also is growing at warp speed. The embryonic hands appear to feel their way toward their correct shape by the presence of the heart.

The limb itself needs to be described. Embryologists in the late 19th century started to consider how to stage embryological development so that they could communicate their findings using agreed criteria. Staging proved to be more difficult than they imagined. G. Streeter developed a staging system in the years 1942 to 1948 (built on by O'Rahilly and Gardner [1975], and O'Rahilly and Müller [1987]). One of the first measurements to be standardized was limb bud length. It was agreed to measure the bud from armpit to tip of the longest digit; this line is known as the ventral axial line. At first this was an imaginary line but it was soon seen to be important for a number of physiological reasons. Early vascular formation coalesces about this mid-ventral line to form an axial artery. Blechschmidt & Gasser (1978) suggest the limbs are biased toward flexion because the flexible but pressurized arteries act as restraining factors (a hydrostatic skeleton) on growth. Another finding confirmed the physiological importance of the limb's ventral midline. Nerves migrate into

CHAPTER 2 • Embryological morphogenesis

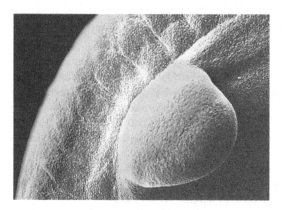

FIG 2.14 **Day 29** The delicate, carefully placed limb bud is clearly emergent. Like the fins of a fish it is placed on the body-wall to control and/or amplify movement. *Reproduced, courtesy of Robert O. Kelley, from Schoenwolf et al 2008, with permission.*

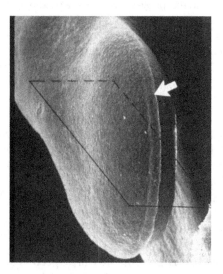

FIG 2.15 **Day 32** The arrow points to the apical ectodermal ridge (AER) of a limb bud. It is a beautiful linear structure. That linearity is hard to attain. Millions of immigrant cells must resolve dorso/ventro and cephalic/caudal tensions to produce a straight line. The AER is essential to normal limb development. It is part of the ectodermal ring that divides the limb bud into the ventral and dorsal domains. The pre-axial border runs along the cephalic ridge of the limb bud. The apical ectodermal ridge (AER) with dorsal (solid) and ventral axial lines is illustrated. The post-axial border at the caudal ridge of the limb bud is also shown. *Reproduced, courtesy of Robert O. Kelley, from Schoenwolf et al 2008, with permission.*

the nascent limb bud via a spiralling penetration that does not cross this midline threshold. Nerves meeting at the ventral axial line are not of adjacent segmental origin, those missing, intervening segments carried down the core of the limb distally (see Fig. 2.16).

The beautiful scanning electron microphotograph in Figure 2.15 shows a limb bud. The arrow points to the AER, which can form only at the junction

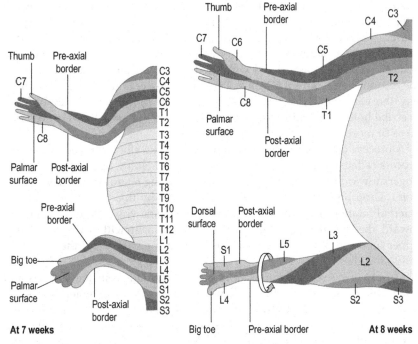

FIG 2.16 **Limb bud rotation** The elbow and knee face laterally at day 50. Over the next 10 days the upper limb is said to externally rotate; the lower limb internally rotates so that the elbow and knee come to approximate each other.

of the ventral and dorsal ectoderm. Many experiments have proved the AER to be essential to normal limb development. Also the microphotograph depicts the ventral axial line (partially hatched) and the dorsal axial line. The existence of the dorsal axial line is routinely depicted in the texts but Keegan and Garrett (1948) question this through their close observation of nerve sensory deficits following compression or section. They propose the pioneer neural cells migrate into the limb bud to meet at the ventral axial line only. Standring (2008), after weighing the evidence, depicts a dorsal axial line as far as the elbow before it breaks up. Here we have 20th-century embryologists discussing the possible significance of an invisible line on the back of an embryonic limb bud.

Two thousand years ago, Chinese medical theorists also considered invisible lines on the midline of the arm. The Pericardium meridian was one of the first to be conceptually established; it is analogous to the ventral axial line. Using associations we can only guess at, the Chinese allocated visceral organs to all the remaining meridians that they came to discern except the arms' dorsal midline. The Chinese must have dithered here as no organs were left unallocated so they created an imaginary organ, the Sanjiao, to associate with the arms' dorsal midline. I find it extraordinary that two cultures, pre-science and bioscience, both pondered invisible lines on the arms and legs, both cultures struggling to understand something fundamental about limb formation, and both having problems with the limbs' dorsal midline.

At the cephalic ridge of the AER the thumb and ring finger will emerge after cells commit suicide – programmed cellular death – to form the finger spaces (Wolpert 2007). The top of the limb bud is called the pre-axial border. Likewise, at the caudal pole of the AER the post-axial border is found. The ventral axial line is associated with the third finger on the upper limb and the second toe (O'Rahilly & Müller 1996) of the lower limb. Note the terminology the early embryologists used in their description of the limb. They describe both lines and borders. Lines are 'strict' whereas borders are often areas of more extensive domainal interaction.

A process called limb bud rotation ensues. The elbow moves caudally, a process called external rotation. If you imagine holding a football with your fingers toward the front, elbows bent and pointing laterally, you have a start point. Drop only your elbows down and feel why this movement is called external rotation. Your chest will tend to widen, and your scapulae will move toward the dorsal body. With further development within the womb the upper limbs become space constrained within the womb and the arms fold across the chest.

Muscle precursor cells migrate into the limb bud from the somites and establish a dorsal and ventral moiety (halves). The ventral moiety gives rise to flexors, pronators, and adductors. The dorsal moiety gives rise to the extensors, supinators, and abductors. These muscle masses then repeatedly split into the definitive muscles of the limb. Meanwhile, cells are streaming into the limb bud from the body wall that is ventral to the Wolffian ridge. This immigrant population will supply the precursor cells of the cartilage and bone. As the cartilage emerges via a condensation effect it sports small tendinous tags. Muscle cells migrate toward and fuse with the tendons in a remarkable example of path finding. How a muscle manages to seek out its appropriate tendon is still unknown (Wolpert 2007). Once the muscles are attached to the tendons the limbs represent a structured union of cells from the dorsal and ventral body. I have often wondered how we might come to understand the Chinese attempt to correlate acupoints on the limbs with visceral function – seeing the limbs as a structured fusion of the dorsal and ventral embryonic body suggests to me that limbs do reflect more than just musculoskeletal biomechanics.

The nerve supply to the muscle moieties reflects this early division into dorsal and ventral muscle. Some muscles migrate from their early position so an embryonic extensor muscle may actually have a flexor action in the adult (such as the brachioradialis). However, the nerve supply is generally considered to be a reliable indicator to the origin of the muscle, be it dorsal or ventral, so the migration of muscle can be tracked.

The development of the lower limb is, in many regards, a similar event to that of the upper limb. Both pairs of limbs emerge from the Wolffian ridge and both specify their primary axes in the same way. However, the hind fins/ limbs have had 500 million years to evolve into their functional niche on the body wall therefore important differences exist. Power generation in most terrestrial vertebrates is analogous to 'rear-wheel drive.' Lower limbs needed to be more massive, which is reflected in how their propulsive drive to the spinal core became hard linked via a large pelvis jointed directly to the spine. Legs are internally rotated (in contrast to the upper limb, which is externally

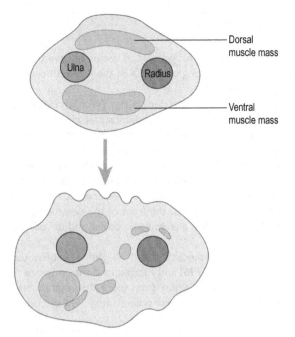

FIG 2.17 **Limb bud muscle moieties** Muscle precursors migrate into the limb bud and form dorsal and ventral moieties. The dorsal moiety forms extensor muscles; the ventral moiety forms flexors. With further development some muscles migrate and assume a different action.

rotated) and, importantly for bipedal hominoids, the lower limb bud is long axis, medially rotated.

If you refer to the limb rotation diagram (see Fig. 2.16) you will see that the elbow and knee are laterally directed. The upper limb externally rotates to bring the elbow inferiorly; the lower limb in contrast internally rotates to bring the knee to face superiorly, combined with the long axis twist that brings the big toes toward each other.

The twisting event in the 7-week-old hind limb involves the very core of the limb as muscle, bone, nerves, and blood vessels are involved. Muscle that was initially on the dorsal aspect of the limb bud is dragged to be ventral in the adult, and vice versa. For this reason it is unwise to link the ventral body-wall to the ventral leg as the ventral body-wall is ventral but the ventral thigh is derived from the dorsal body via leg rotation.

Limb development

■ In general, but not in every detail, development takes place in a proximal/distal direction. For example, the portions of the limb bud that will be the shoulder manifest before the hand portions.
■ The primitive mesoderm that will form the limb bud is influenced and induced proximally by the intermediate mesoderm, i.e. urogenital

development and the coelom. Again TCM seems to have pre-dated this insight by 2000 years, insisting on the Qi of the kidneys being essential for limb growth and strength.

■ Limb buds emerge from the ectodermal ring (Wolffian ridge) so their genesis is intimately connected to the developmental cascades that induce the nose, eyes, ears, nipples, and genital tip. The finger/toe tips are analogous to the tip of your genitalia in their neurological sensitivity.

■ Immigrant early bone and muscle cells establish themselves in dorso/ventro and pre-/post-axial domains. With limb bud development this pattern is modified. The hind limb musculature becomes coiled. Muscle that was at the back of the limb bud migrates to the front of the developing leg. In effect the leg musculature acts like a pogo stick, coiling and uncoiling in our gait pattern.

■ At full term the spine is flexed, the head is slightly side bent, usually to the right (O'Rahilly & Müller 1996) and rotated, and the limbs are tightly flexed (the foot has so much dorsiflexion it can touch the ventral tibia via squatting facets). Squatting is a deeply human posture that I will discuss at length later in the text.

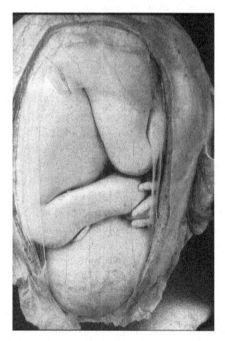

FIG 2.18 **Photograph of a full-term embryo** Note the tightly flexed posture. At full term the ankles are fully dorsiflexed so that the foot can touch the shin. *From England 1990.*

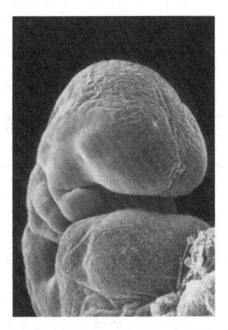

FIG 2.19 **Week four** At this stage in development the brain and the heart nearly touch. The maxillary and the mandibular processes are derived from the first pharyngeal arch. The second and third pharyngeal arches are visible behind the massive heart. *Reproduced, courtesy of A. Tamarin, from Schoenwolf et al 2008.*

THE FACE

The face emerges between the brain and the heart – our thoughts and our feelings.

The mammalian face is the most expressive on the animal planet. The brain comes to the surface at the eyes, the mouth represents the opening to the entire gut system, whilst muscles, ranging from the strongest to the most delicate, animate our feelings. The face has five primary centers of growth, often called 'processes,' that coalesce to form the most morphologically complex region of the body's external form.

At 4 weeks post conception the anterior brain is seen with a scanning electron microscope as a large frontonasal process. The brain is developing at warp speed, stretching the dural membranes that contain and compartmentalize it. At this stage it is externally featureless as there are no sense organs. Below the brain is a closed-off cavity, the stomodeum, that will be the future mouth. Both lateral and below the stomodeum are the early manifestations of the upper and lower jaw. These bilateral structures, the maxillary and the mandibular processes, are derived from a structure called the first pharyngeal arch. Thus the face will emerge from the interaction of the frontonasal process and the bilateral processes that contribute to the jaw apparatus, derived from the first pharyngeal arch. Humans have five pharyngeal arches that are small folds of tissue below the brain. The pharyngeal arches differentiate into much of the face and throat region.

The first hint of a nose appears as two discs called (olfactory) placodes on the lateral sides of the frontonasal process. Only animals with a brain encased in a cranium develop placodes. The placodes are thickened ectodermal discs that appear on the surface of the brain. Placodes are in some ways similar to the previously introduced AER of the limb buds. The Wolffian ridge courses over the AER of the limb buds and, in the throat/face region, encompasses the various placodes that manifest there. Placodes contribute to the olfactory sensory epithelium, the lens of the eyes, and the inner ear. The olfactory placodes are related in vertebrates to the very front of the forebrain, a region called the rhinencephalon. In humans, this region of the brain has diminished in size, being relegated to an inconspicuous anteroventral location, but in the fishes it is as large as the cerebral hemispheres that emerge just behind. The placodes appear on the surface of the brain, then ingress, vortex like, toward the forebrain, forming a ring of tissue around what are now called nasal pits. The left and right nasal pits are surrounded by medial and lateral nasal prominences that are drawn toward the midline where they fuse together to form a recognizable nose and philtrum.

Lateral to the nasal pits are the two optic placodes. Many vertebrates below birds also have a functional third eye at the top of the head. This photoreceptor does not form a visual image but registers the duration and intensity of solar radiation, which is used to help regulate physiology. The bilateral optic placodes form the optic pits that are drawn down under the skin to then transform into the lenses of the eyes. The lens is surrounded by an island of the central nervous system (CNS) that is connected directly to the brain by the optic nerve. Many upstream genes cooperate to induce developmental cascades that form these complex sense organs (Carroll 2005).

Still further laterally and caudally, the first sign of the ears are the otic placodes that are associated with the hindbrain. Once again, the placodes invaginate to form the otic pits that will close over to create the otic vesicles, which in turn morph to become the inner ear. Meanwhile, the external ear is formed from six little auricular hillocks that line the first and second pharyngeal arch. Three hillocks that are astride the lower jaw which is part of the first pharyngeal arch merge and complexly morph with the three hillocks from the second pharyngeal arch. Only mammals have external ears (also called the auricle or pinna). As described below, the second pharyngeal arch will also contribute the muscles of facial expression and the top half of the hyoid bone.

Placodes not only contribute to the formation of the nose, eye, and ear, but other placodes that overlay the pharyngeal arches, probably derived from the lateral line system of fish, contribute to sensation from the face, tongue, throat, and viscera. Their role in embryonic development is crucial. Placodes metaphorically appear to be like buoys that the brain floats to the surface of the embryo to correctly position itself in development with two buoys to the front (nasal), two buoys to the sides (otic), and two buoys to the intermediate region (optic). Then the brain draws the buoys back to itself to cement that positional status. Again the importance of the Wolffian ridge to development is apparent as all the placodes, the limb buds, the nipples, and the genitals are encompassed by that transient structure.

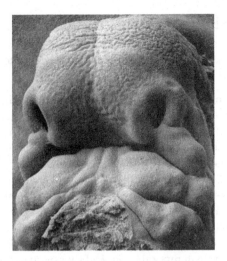

FIG 2.20 **Week six** The nasal placodes have invaginated leaving the nasal pits surrounded by the medial and lateral nasal prominences. The maxillary process has developed just below the nasal prominences. Eventually it will join its contralateral fellow. Below is the mandibular process with three auricular hillocks that, with another three from the second pharyngeal arch, will coalesce to form the external ear. *Reproduced, courtesy of A. Tamarin, from Schoenwolf et al 2008.*

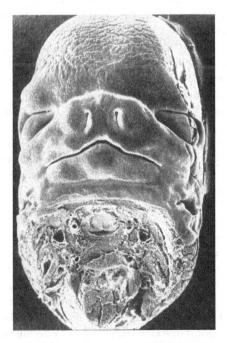

FIG 2.21 **Week seven** The eyes that were more lateral have been drawn toward the front. The nose is now clearly discernable, as are the upper and lower jaw. *Reproduced, courtesy of A. Tamarin, from Schoenwolf et al 2008.*

THE PHARYNGEAL ARCHES

The pharyngeal arches are derived from the gill apparatus of ancient fish. The nerves and muscles that move the gills of a fish have, in humans, been appropriated for listening and winking, talking and swallowing.

Before the embryonic folding event the heart precursor tissue sits above the brain. With folding the heart moves ventrally down the 'throat' region toward the 'chest' region. The rapidly growing brain requires the heart to keep up the circulation to billions of new cells. Between the brain bending forward and the heart thrusting upward, the tissue of the 'neck' region pleats into small but distinct structures called the pharyngeal arches, homologous to the gills of fish. The five human pharyngeal arches that appear do so in a cranio-caudal sequence. Each arch is associated with a cranial nerve, a blood vessel, and musculoskeletal elements.

As outlined above the first pharyngeal arch will form the upper and lower jaw, zygoma, part of the temporal bone, and two small ear bones, the malleus and the incus. The mammalian ear is unique in that it has three bones involved in the conduction of sound. The nerve associated with this arch is the trigeminal – cranial nerve V. Muscles derived from the first arch are the muscles of mastication (the temporalis, masseter, pterygoids), and a couple of small muscles of the ear.

The second pharyngeal arch contributes to the stapes of the ear, the styloid process, and part of the hyoid bone. A shark, in contrast, without three bones in its ear, uses bones derived from this arch to extend its jaw when it is about to bite. Our enhanced ability to hear is related to fewer bones involved in the biting apparatus. Muscles from this arch migrate up to the face to form the numerous muscles of facial expression, all innervated by the facial nerve – cranial VII. In the neurological hierarchy these muscles reside just caudal to the muscles of mastication.

Pharyngeal arches three, four, and six (arch five is rudimentary and disappears) form part of the hyoid, and the laryngeal cartilages. Muscles derived from these arches constrict the pharynx and operate the larynx. A shark uses these arches to support and operate the gills; we use them to talk, swallow, and turn the head (Shubin 2008). Nerves associated with these arches are the glossopharyngeal (cranial IX), and the vagus (X).

SUMMARY

Embryology is often perceived by students to be of little practical use, too hard to come to terms with, and hence one of the most unpopular courses taught at medical, physiotherapy, and osteopathy degrees. Anatomy of adult structures may be quite different in early development, and words struggle to depict what is happening rapidly in three dimensions. But it is an essential context to have in place if one is to come to grips with human form and function. The contractile field model both draws on, and pays homage to, this context. Key events described here include cleavage, compaction, gastrulation and the embryonic disc, folding, the coelom, the Wolffian ridge, limb buds, the face, and the pharyngeal arches. Do not expect to get your head around embryology on the first reading. Rather it is like a mosaic that takes time to construct as information from various sources comes together to gradually form a coherent picture.

REFERENCES

Blechschmidt E, Gasser R 1978 Biokinetics and biodynamics of human differentiation. Thomas, Illinois

Bloom TL 1989 The effects of phorbol ester on mouse blastomeres. Development 106:159–171

Carlson B 1994 Human embryology and developmental biology. Mosby, St Louis

Carlson B 2009 Human embryology and developmental biology, 4th edn. Mosby, St Louis

Carroll S 2005 Endless forms most beautiful. Weidenfeld & Nicolson, London

England M 1990 A colour atlas of life before birth. Mosby Year Books, Philadelphia

Fitzgerald M, Fitzgerald M 1978 Human embryology. Harper & Row, London

Gilbert S 1997 Developmental biology, 5th edn. Sinauer Associates Inc, Sunderland

Kardong K 1998 Vertebrates: comparative anatomy, function, evolution, 2nd edn. WCB/McGraw-Hill, Boston, p 51

Keegan J, Garrett F 1948 The segmental distribution of the cutaneous nerves in the limbs of man. The Anatomical Record (102):409–437

Kelley R 1985 Early development of the vertebrate limb: an introduction to morphogenetic tissue interaction using scanning electron microscopy. Scanning Electron Microscopy 11:827–836

Larsen W 1993 Human embryology. Churchill Livingstone, New York

O'Rahilly R, Gardner E 1975 The timing and sequence of events in the development of the limbs in the human embryo. Anatomy and Embryology 148:1–23

O'Rahilly R, Müller F 1985 The origins of the ectodermal ring in staged human embryology. Acta Anatomica 122:145–157.

O'Rahilly R, Müller F 1987 Developmental stages in human embryos. Carnegie Institution, Washington

O'Rahilly R, Müller F 1996 Human embryology & teratology, 2nd edn. Wiley-Liss, New York

Raff R 1996 The shape of life. University of Chicago Press, Chicago

Sandler T 1990 Langman's medical embryology. Williams & Wilkins, Baltimore

Schoenwolf G, Bleyl S, Brauer P et al 2008 Larsen's human embryology, 4th edn. Churchill Livingstone, New York

Shubin N 2008 Your inner fish; a journey into the 3.5 billion-year history of the human body. Allen Lane, London

Standring S 2008 Gray's anatomy, 40th edn. Churchill Livingstone, Philadelphia

Stephens T 1982 The Wolffian ridge: history of a misconception. Isis 73(267):254–257

Wendell C, Williams P 1984 Basic human embryology. Pitman, London

Wolpert L 1991 The triumph of the embryo. Oxford University Press, Oxford

Wolpert L 2007 Principles of development, 3rd edn. Oxford University Press, Oxford

Modelling movement

3

Much of the modern approach to the understanding of musculoskeletal ease and dis-ease is predicated on a cadaveric approach to anatomy. In contrast, an emphasis on a whole organism approach to functional anatomy will suggest new assessment methodologies, and inform diverse approaches to rehabilitation.

Shakespeare's play *As You Like It* (1600) contains these classic lines:

Rosalind: But are you so much in love as your rhymes speak?

Orlando: Neither rhyme nor reason can express how much.

This chapter looks at the rhyme and reason that informs the contractile field (CF) model. By rhyme I mean the use of analogy and metaphor that so richly infuses the biological sciences. Analogy is the correspondence or adaptation of one thing (the source) to another (the target), for example a *New Scientist* magazine article was headed 'Save the Economy – Treat it Like a Polluted Swamp' (Mackenzie 2008). The use of analogy aids the transfer of information from one known domain to another. It acts as a gel-like mediator that morphs to convey meaning or essence from source to target. Analogy does not offer a proof but it aids high-level perception. In the biological sense, structures are analogous when they perform similar functions but are derived from different evolutionary pathways. Hence the wing of a fly is said to be analogous to the human forelimb but it is homologous to (i.e. has shared ancestry with) the wing of a bird.

The essence of metaphor is understanding and experiencing one kind of thing in terms of another. The word is derived from the Greek 'to transfer' or 'carry across' (Lakoff & Johnson 1980). The use of metaphor is intrinsic to language; it is unavoidable, ubiquitous, and mostly unconscious. Metaphors are fundamentally conceptual in nature yet are grounded in everyday experience. Whether we recognize it or not our choice of analogy and metaphor profoundly influences the way we come to develop an understanding of a topic. For example, consider the human brain. We tend to think in terms of

53

© 2010 Elsevier Ltd / Inc / Bv
DOI: 10.1016/B978-0-7020-3109-0.00008-0

neural switches, pathways, regions lit up when active, or complex circuits that route information. Gerald Edelman (1992) suggests the individual human brain is more like a unique and unimaginably dense rainforest, teeming with growth and decay. It is less like a programmed machine than an ecological habitat that mimics the evolution of life itself. The brain as a bio-computer or a rainforest induces starkly contrasting associations that profoundly influence the way we relate to the subject.

Daniel Kahneman (2008), a psychologist at Princeton University (a recipient of the 2002 Nobel Prize in Economics) has been working on the way the brain creates and employs these associative networks. Advances in technology have allowed the brain's reaction times to words to be accurately measured. Words flashing onto a computer screen 'prime' a vast associative network in the subject's brain, much of it subliminal but real in its effect on behavior. Kahneman describes how the word 'vomit' flashed for less than a second will cause facial gestures, a withdrawal from the computer screen and a priming of an associative structure that emerges from exposure to the word. Hundreds of words that you associate with vomit are now primed and more reactive as evidenced by faster reaction times. So likewise the word 'rainforest' will initiate a cascade of associative thought that will color the direction of subsequent enquiry. The analogy and metaphors we use when introducing a new idea are not linguistic flourishes but rather are crucial associative aids needed to develop conceptual pathways and high-order understandings.

The reason in 'rhyme and reason' means to think out, to arrange the thought of, in a logical and verifiable manner. Reason is a conscious attempt to discover what is true and best, with notions of cause and effect derived from first principles. However, life is intrinsically so parsimonious yet so flamboyant, reducible yet irreducible, so complexly layered and messy that the conscious blending of both rhyme and reason offers our best chance to forge a way forward.

A model is a tentative ideational structure used as a testing device. It is tentative because the model is not the system under study, just as the map is not the terrain. It is ideational because it exists in the realm of the mind, so much so that model building can almost be a definition of mind. Minds create models as abstractions from reality in that they emphasize only a few parts so that the great complexity in worldly relations may be more clearly perceived. Models are generated from the close observation of large systems. Detail is selectively shed revealing the primary building blocks, the crucial components of the system that through their interaction produce emergent qualities similar to those of the observed system. The trick is to know what to keep and what to shed as one reaches tentatively toward the essentials of the observed system.

John Holland (1998), author of *Emergence – From Chaos to Order*, discusses a tension within successful modelling, a tension between the generality which the shearing away of detail gives v. the pointedness of experimental analysis. He suggests analogy, metaphor, and intuition, often via an interdisciplinary weaving, are essential to model construction. To select the primary building blocks of a large system requires one to be immersed in the discipline for many years, alert to nuance and relationship. To develop a model, both rhyme and reason need to be employed.

Models yield predictions, allow planning, reveal possibilities and consequences, and aid the discernment of critical phenomena such as bifurcation and system control points (Morgan & Morrison 1999). This is why we model, and why the value of models to us is profound. Importantly, learning from models occurs at two places – in their construction and then in their use.

Most of the professions that this book targets carry out their professional practice on whole, living people. We do not have a surgical mandate. However, our anatomical knowledge base is derived in large part from the careful dissection of cadavers. Individual muscles are dissected out and we then imagine that muscle acting in isolation moving a body part. Yet in everyday living reality, when a person arises from the floor and turns to greet you, hundreds of muscles acting from eye to toe will have been used in an exquisitely choreographed temporal sequence. To better understand whole organism movement patterns we need to develop models that aid our understanding at that level of the biological hierarchy. For too long we have used the dissective paradigm abstracted from the dead body to understand living musculoskeletal ease and dis-ease. The clinical results derived from this mismatch have been disappointing.

We use this dissective paradigm to diagnose and to then inform our modes of treatment. An orthopedic-style musculoskeletal examination is predicated on the dissective paradigm. Each 'test,' usually 'challenging' of a tissue, is directed toward naming the tissue at fault. For example, a small muscle of the back, say the multifidus, or a named joint, say the sacroiliac, is said to be responsible for the patient's low back pain. That named muscle or joint will then be the focus for treatment. However, it is proving to be notoriously difficult to realistically arrive at a tissue causing symptoms diagnosis for syndromes such as low back pain, or headaches, or knee pain, etc. When the symptomatology is more complex, chronic, and diffuse the quest to arrive at a precise diagnosis is often inconclusive. Symptoms can be fickle as they often change in location and character, even over brief time periods. Quite severe symptoms can emerge with no apparent structural cause, and vice versa, frank musculoskeletal derangement may not be associated with pain or distress (Jensen et al 1994). The named tissue may well be structurally and functionally compromised but that named tissue is part of a matrix; it is often a fall guy for a discordance that runs through large areas of the living body. For example, a population of the patients seeking treatment for a musculoskeletal disorder in New Zealand had almost 78% simply classified as being regional pain disorders or back pain (Taylor et al 2004).

We use the dissective paradigm when we go to the gym. After sitting all day we sit on a 'pec deck,' or a 'lat pulldown' machine to work a named muscle to exhaustion. When in life do we need to sit, reach up and behind us to then repeatedly pull a heavy weight that is stabilized in all directions except up/down? Exercises predicated on isolated muscles look bizarre to the uninitiated. Gyms used to be called barbell clubs during the era of the strong man (around 1900–1960), with records for competitive lifts such as the 'two hand anyhow' (Arthur Saxon) that have remained unbroken for over a century. There must be very few sports that still have an unbroken record despite a now global participation using sophisticated sports training methods, and too often drugs. It would seem the trend toward machine-based exercises has not produced the functional strength needed for a complex lift such as the 'two hand anyhow.'

Muscles groomed via a machine that isolates major groups may look good (if big is good) in the mirror but muscles pumped through this selective isolation are often surprisingly functionally inefficient in the non-gym context. Some years ago I trekked in Nepal. One of my fellow walkers was a pumped-up gym man who after a few days decided to carry a female porter's 45 kg load for half a day. The next day this chap could hardly move, which made the porters very happy. Resource transport has been an intrinsic part of the tool-using human condition for millions of years. Floor sitting to standing, walking, running, and transporting resources is a developmental continuum that sitting at a 'lat pulldown' machine will just not address.

Seeing movement as whole organism fields of contractility that have evolved along functional pathways that we increasingly understand offers us fresh approaches to assessment and treatment of the moving body.

FIELDS

Joseph Needham proposed that '[A] field ... is a dynamic description of a spatio-temporal activity, not a mere geometrical picture of a momentary time-slice in the organism's history' (Needham 1936, p. 108). He was part of a small but intensely motivated group of theoretical biologists working on animal development in the 1930s. Science had begun a mapping of the universe and was about to split the atom. Physics was breathtaking in its new powers of creation and destruction – it was the dominant science. Biology, in contrast, was struggling. The world of animals was so unruly, so diverse and often perverse, that biologists struggled to make sense of what they became privy to. For example, the scientific exploration of embryology opened a window into a world, a world of extraordinary form generation and transformation that had been, until microscopes, only fleetingly accessible in hallucinogenic states. How did form arise and transform, that from the first is a living functionality, in a state of incandescent becoming? Scientists could watch and marvel but they had few explanatory insights. In 1931 Needham wrote a three-volume *Chemical Embryology* series published by Cambridge University Press, his career seemingly at a peak. In 1937 a brilliant young Chinese student, Lu Gwei-djen, travelled from China to study with Needham and his wife Dorothy, who was also a scientist specializing in muscle physiology. A relationship was established that changed their lives and lasted a lifetime. Needham learnt Chinese language and became a vocal advocate for many of the socio-political issues of the day that affected China and the UK. Japan invaded China in July 1937, with particularly vicious attacks on Chinese centers of higher education. Needham became very involved, so much so he was to spend the World War II years in non-occupied China on behalf of the English government offering succour to what was left of their academia (Winchester 2008). Here he realized the enormous depth of early Chinese science as his voracious mind observed and absorbed all manner of science and technology about him. He perceived there a mode of thinking that resonated with his own.

Out of these experiences was to come one of the world's greatest academic series, the near mythical 'Science and Civilisation in China', now up to 24 parts of which 17 were published under his direct supervision.

Needham was thinking about biological fields because of his embryological studies. Years of peering down microscopes, watching and manipulating morphogenesis, had convinced him that interacting fields underlie the genesis of form and could explain much of what he saw. Contemporary theoretical biology is still thinking about fields, probably because they are so ubiquitous. O'Rahilly and Müller (1996), two of the world's foremost authorities on the human embryo, state:

The subdivision of the embryonic body into fields precedes the formation of specific organs or structures. (p. 93)

Fields are intrinsically dynamic systems and structures that have robust properties that accommodate normal and abnormal variance. They can exhibit the ability to divide and fuse, push and pull, corrode, shear, invaginate, induce, contract, or blossom. Fields can profoundly interact or show relative independence from other fields, that interaction changing over time. Hierarchies of fields within fields are the norm.

During the embryonic period, pioneer muscle tissue rides on migratory pathways that look like accelerated weather systems. These morphogenetic fields – fields that create shape and organization – have polarities and borders. In some respects they exhibit fluid-like behavior with the flow of ocean currents layering and twisting being a suitable metaphor. Somehow, muscle fiber direction, depth, and continuity are instilled in the primordial muscle tissue during this early migration.

Core patterns of contractility, allied to field-like behavior, suggest new ways to understand human movement. Contractility will be expected to widen and narrow as it courses about the body. When it widens the speed of movement slows and spreads like a wide, shallow river. When contractility narrows toward an insertion it will speed up and focus force. Like the warp and weft of a complex textile, it is obligatory that contractility will rise toward superficial fascial layers then dive toward deep layers and the endoskeleton. Fields of contractility will also demonstrate the ability to twist. A sheet of contractile tissue may twist so that what was a superficial surface when twisted becomes a deep surface. When two or more contractile sheets are twisted together they will fuse fiber directions to form a dense nodal region that is knot-like, for example the perineal body of the pelvic floor.

The coursing of contractility is most evident in the embryonic period when genetic cascades and morphogenetic fields interact on a system-wide scale, but the most stable of the developmental processes is that of the adult, hence it is of special significance. Goodwin (1994) emphasizes the conceptual importance of the biology of whole organisms when he states:

I take the position that organisms are as real, as fundamental, as irreducible, as the molecules out of which they are made. They are a separate and distinct level of emergent biological order, and the one to which we most immediately relate since we ourselves are organisms. (p. xii)

All professions that deal with the order and disorder of human movement need to regain context by stepping back and revaluing the whole organism perspective. To do this we need to use field theory and develop models as mediators.

Over the past 50 years, various authors have proposed linking muscles together into cohesive patterns (see Busquet 1992, Dart 1950, Godelieve 1995). The musculature is so complex it is easy to link one myofascial structure to another, but without a whole organism perspective derived from dearly held vertebrate constructional norms, the act of drawing lines about the body is of little use. The many lines that traverse the body depicted by Busquet (1992) fall into this trap (as contrasted with Dart, who was professorial across anatomy, evolutionary anthropology, and human movement via his studies with FM Alexander). Furthermore, to use dissective studies to validate how muscles interact across the body to form patterns of movement is a process that is fraught with difficulty. It is just too easy to simply select lines of tissue association and dissect out what does not fit. A cross-section through the neck will reveal muscles running in every fiber direction from longitudinal to transverse – pick the fiber direction one wants to keep and dissect the rest away. Dissective studies that do this are of little value. Dissectional studies must first and foremost be derived from the selection of the building blocks of the model, and then the clear application of the methodology to the cadaver.

Of the literature on the subject that I am familiar with, only Thomas Myers (2009) has developed a model of human movement that is a serious attempt to map global myofascial patterns, a process he calls the Anatomy Trains. He describes 'myofascial meridians' via a train line metaphor that uses images such as stations, tracks, and switches to describe myofascial continuity. It is a considerably different approach to the difficult problem of modelling movement.

Firstly, the metaphoric language used is in contrast to that used in the CF model. In the CF model there are no trains, stations, or rail tracks in the biological world. Rather fields, cascades, migrations, fluid dynamics, etc. are more likely to provide the sources that will generate the analogy and metaphor used in this study. Secondly, his model is based on direct myofascial connections whereas the CF model does not confine itself in this way. Fascia envelops everything so the term myofascial, an ever broader term, actually means very little. Both muscle and fascia are mainly derived from the middle of the three embryonic layers (mesoderm), but so too are the kidneys and blood. There is no need to impose on the body a rule that demands direct myofascial connections to construct a model of movement; in fact I suggest it detracts from a deeper analysis. Thirdly, the Anatomy Train model falls into the trap of linking ventral torso musculature to ventral leg musculature, whereas the embryology does not suggest this, as detailed in Chapter 3 of this book. Good models are transferable; they can be employed to cross-domains. How would a model like the Anatomy Trains cope with a vertebrate such as a snake that has lost its limbs during evolutionary development? For conceptual clarity it is best to consider the limbs as fields in their own right, fields that are in turn, nested within larger morphogenic fields. Fourthly, external body-wall and limb musculature is only the shell of a movement model if conceptual space is not given to the kidneys and the visceral musculature.

Interested readers should study both models, but do keep in mind these are amongst the first attempts to model whole organism movement patterning so over the next couple of decades they will be vastly improved upon. We accept that modelling the economy or climate is only ever approximate; so too is the modelling of human movement.

SYSTEMS THEORY

The CF model draws on systems theory to help provide a conceptual framework. Systems theory is an attempt to discover what features are common to all systems (McKenzie & James 2004). A system is defined as something that maintains its existence and functions as a whole through the interaction of its parts (O'Connor & McDermott 1997). Systems exhibit dynamic complexity where the elements of a system can relate in many different ways. Systems are not end to end but rather nested so that there are subordinate and superordinate relationships. Relationships between systems and components within a system have boundaries but within those boundaries there is considerable space for novelty.

To gain influence over a system it is necessary to understand the structure of the system. Systems have nodal regions where the levers of control manifest. Input to a system will often have a time delay before the system responds, and that response may be far away in the system. Time lag, non-local effects, and unexpected side-effects are intrinsic to systems. Because systems are all about component interaction when you are dealing with a system you can never do just one thing. Like a strong net, systems tend to self-correct and self-stabilize unless crucial nodal regions and relationships are compromised.

EMERGENCE

The concept of emergence is at once both simple and profound. Emergence is the quality described when we say the whole is greater than the sum of its parts. Goldstein (1999) suggests 'the arising of novel and coherent structures, patterns, and properties during the process of self-organization in complex systems' (p. 49) defines emergence. Johnson (2001) suggests coming to terms with emergence lies in the accumulation of descriptive models. Systems theory and emergence are closely related. Both concepts are constrained by rules and the interaction of components. Board games have been used to explore the nature of emergence. For example, chess is defined by about 20 rules, but after hundreds of years of intense study we are still finding new possibilities in the game. Only after exhaustive study did we discern some of the deep patterns that are embedded in the game of chess (Holland 1998). Using pawn formations and sacrificial gambits allowed players to become more powerful and controlling of the flow of the game. A similar analogy would be the martial arts. After millions of years of just bashing the opponent with brute savagery, effective techniques of offense and defense emerged. What we are finding is how surprisingly rich and transcendent emergent properties can be, and how useful. Much of our modern technological life is derived from employing emergence – think fine wine, beer, and cheese.

I hypothesize the meridians of Traditional Chinese Medicine (TCM) are emergent lines of shape control. Chinese culture over thousands of years studied human shape in both health and disease to discern an underlying pattern that only now, with modern neurobiology, are we able to re-comprehend. The latter part of this book will develop this hypothesis.

SENSE ORGANS – EMBEDDED

Recently, at a restaurant, I saw a woman have a violent epileptic attack. Movement without control is destructive and dangerous. Vertebrates, via their body-plan, have wired their sense organs, their central nervous systems, and their moving bodies together. You cannot call yourself a vertebrate if your ears originate in front of your nose. The vertebrate brain is wired to the deeply conserved pattern of olfaction in front, vision intermediate, and auditory/balance senses behind and lateral on the sensory platform of the head. Change this layout and be prepared to change the fundamental architecture that links our sense organs to our brain, and our brain to our movement patterns – patterns of association that vertebrates have used to move volitionally for 500 million years.

The Chinese meridial map suggested this important associative pattern to me. If the nerve that emanates from each spinal segment is analogous to local government then the sense organs are analogous to central government. When I suggest the olfactory organs are embedded in the dorso/ventro-contractile field (D/V-CF) I do not imply that they inform only movement in the dorso/ventro plane. Rather, it is suggested that during early embryogenesis, the morphogenic fields that course around the embryo on either side of the dorsal and ventral midline also course over the embryonic nasal placodes that are the first external manifestations of the future nose. Placodes for the nose, eyes, and ears may act as buoys or lighthouses that help morphogenesis proceed correctly. Embedding sense organs (or other nodal tissues) in specific CFs is novel, suggests avenues of enquiry, and is conceptually elegant.

THE CONTRACTILE FIELDS – AN OVERVIEW

The Spinal Engine by Serge Gracovetsky (1988) is an examination of the biomechanics of the lumbar spine. Gracovetsky used a cartoon character called a 'critter' to demonstrate the key movements employed by a tetrapod in its gait pattern. He used an evolutionary approach that succinctly captured the role of the lumbar spine in our bipedal gait pattern. Gracovetsky illustrated the critter side-bending, rotating, flexing, and extending, and then coupling these movements to torque the spine.

Each of the CFs that I will now preview act as an intrinsic part of a whole. Separating the fields is an intellectual abstraction that aids the comprehension of our complex musculature; the fields do not exist of themselves. The pattern of relationship between the CFs is as important as the fields themselves. We move as a whole organism, seamlessly blending the primal movement patterns I describe in this book. These movement patterns consist of the:

- Dorso/ventro contractile field (D/V-CF)
- Lateral contractile field (L-CF)

- Helical contractile field (H-CF), which emerges from the interaction of the D/V-CF and the L-CF
- Limb contractile fields (Limb-CFs) with dorsal and ventral moieties
- Radial contractile field (R-CF)
- Fluid field (F-F)
- Chiralic contractile fields (C-CFs), which have pulsatile and peristaltic functions.

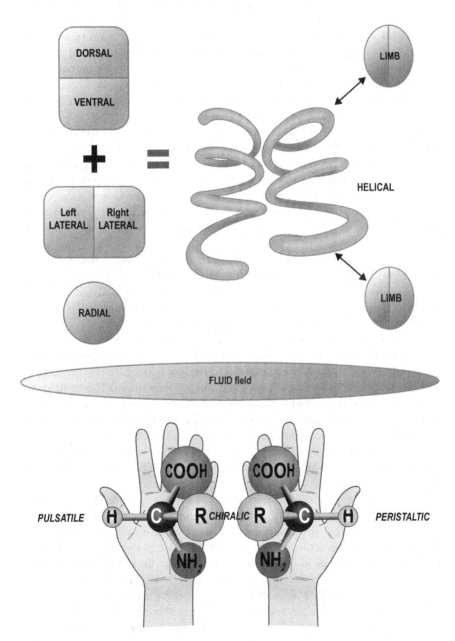

FIG 3.1   A schema of the contractile fields model Lower part courtesy of NASA Astrobiology Institute.

We start with a lateral CF (L-CF), as bending to the side is a core movement pattern that can be traced back to early fish (Long 1995). The L-CF is modelled as being a bilaminar sheet of contractility that courses up from the perineal body, up the sides of the torso, left/right crosses (decuss) at the sub-occipital region, and then courses over the embedded otic (ear) region to then turn toward the lateral rectus muscle of the eyeball. The L-CF is like a figure 8 with the cross points being the pelvic floor, the sub-occipital region, and the ears/lateral eyes.

Between the left and right lateral musculature of the L-CF lies the dorso/ventro CF (D/V-CF). Rivers of contractility course on either side of both the dorsal and ventral midline to encircle the body from the rostral (toward the nose) apex of the head to the pelvic floor. The left and right rings of contractility are not isolated from each other as they are twisted together when coursing through the pelvic floor and the sub-occipital region. The D/V-CF musculature creates a seamless, twisted, paraxial ring of contractility, with the olfactory organs embedded in this field.

We now need to consider how a biomechanical combination of the L-CF and the D/V-CF creates a torque of the spine, called in this model the helical contractile field (H-CF). A helix can be left- or right-handed. When looking along the axis of a helix, if a clockwise movement moves one away from the observer it is a right-handed helix, and vice versa. Our species has specialized in this helical field of contractility because we have employed it in our bipedal gait pattern and in our ability to over-arm throw.

The H-CF is envisaged as an encircling river of contractility that is characterized by fascial depth change and neurological left/right switching as it repeatedly crosses the ventral and dorsal midline. It will conceptually originate from the tip of the genitals to then coil its way around the body to terminate at the eyes, the embedded sense organ for this field.

Flexion or extension, lateral flexion, and twisting left or right, if carried too far will buckle and injure the spinal system. Buckling or kinking the spine is a painful event that takes many months to recover from, thus it is imperative that the length of the spine is preserved during movement. The radial contractile field (R-CF) has a squeezing effect on the body-wall that elongates the spinal system, as imagined by a torso-shaped tube of plasticine, which when squeezed about the circumference, will elongate but narrow. The R-CF will thus squeeze the torso, or the opposite movement, which is to suck. All mammals suckle with uniquely mobile lips so this CF embeds the lips and the external anal ring at the caudal end of the gut tube.

Limbs emerge as small buds from the body-wall of the 24–26-day-old embryo. They develop quickly so that at birth they are large structures that go on growing to become a large percentage of our adult body length and mass. The limb contractile fields (Limb-CFs) are simply modelled as having a ventral and a dorsal muscle mass (also called moieties, meaning halves) to which all the limb bones and muscles can be hypothetically traced back. Limbs are also modelled as emerging from specific sites on the embryonic body-wall that I suggest are associated with helical biodynamics. Limbs plug into and empower the H-CF in particular. The hands and feet are the embedded sense organs for Limb-CFs.

It soon becomes apparent in the modelling process that the body-wall and limb musculature are only a partial descriptor of movement. Intermediate mesoderm forms the kidneys and aspects of the genital system. A fluid field (F-F) is hypothesized that acts via the kidneys to maintain, within narrow physiological norms, interstitial fluid throughout the body. Both embryology and comparative evolutionary anatomy point to a deeply held association between the coelom and kidney physiology. In the early stages of development the coelomic fluid both surrounds the embryo and courses within it. Fluids of many named types are communicating with each other via pressure gradients. Later in life, a world-class athlete will come to a grinding halt if a strong diuretic drug disrupts the delicate fluid balances within the body. Fluid dynamics are so essential to life and the propagation of life itself, that to construct a model of movement without acknowledging the centrality of the fluid specialist mesodermal organ – the kidneys – would be to miss a key part of this complex summation we call movement.

Lateral to the intermediate mesoderm, contractile tissue flows into two leaves, the outer forming the body-wall/limbs, the inner forming a leaf called the splanchnic mesoderm – it contributes to the visceral and cardiogenic musculature. The cardinal difference between body-wall musculature and visceral musculature I model as being the difference between symmetry and asymmetry. All the muscles of the body-wall and limbs are bilaterally symmetrical. The word 'chiralic,' as it is used here, describes the non-symmetric but handed nature of the visceral muscle. Between the symmetric and the asymmetric lies the coelom and the kidneys. The C-CF explicitly acknowledges the crucial role of the cardiovascular system (pulsatile) and the gastrointestinal system (peristaltic) in our ability to move.

ARCHETYPAL POSTURES

The CF model is a whole-system approach to human movement. The following chapters will detail each CF. Assessment protocols derived from a cadaveric approach to anatomy will be in large part inappropriate for this model. How does one then assess whole person movement patterns?

Movement is the coherent changing of shape – some shapes we assume are more fundamental than others. Like the notes that underlie music, I suggest that some postures, particularly floor-based postures of repose, tune our bodies. Rest is to movement as the heart's diastolic blood pressure is to the heart's systolic blood pressure. We need to consider both sides of the coin, that is, both rest and movement, if we are to advance the understanding of the human biomechanical condition. The concept of tune as used in this book is developed in Chapter 11.

DECODING THE CHINESE MERIDIAL MAP

Both the CF model and the archetypal postures are then employed to take a fresh look at the enigmatic meridians of TCM. The Chinese people used an associative and synthetic approach to their way of making sense of the world about them. If meridians do have more intrinsic meaning than just an aide-memoire for linking random trigger points, the decoding I hypothesize is

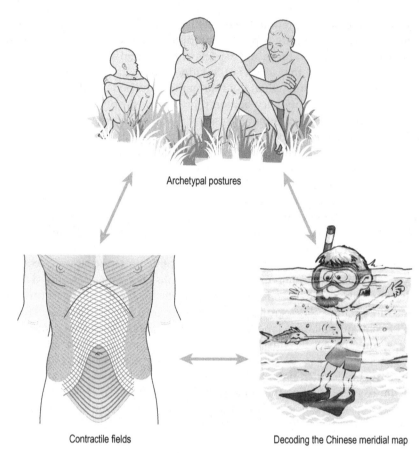

Archetypal postures

Contractile fields

Decoding the Chinese meridial map

FIG 3.2 **Three primary areas of interest constitute this book** *Original cartoon drawing by MONSTAcartoons (Mark O'Brien). © Elsevier.*

worthy of investigation. It uses a methodology the Chinese would have had access to, which is manual therapy handholds, allied with how we move instinctively away from a penetrating or otherwise painful event.

REFERENCES

Busquet L 1992 Les chaînes musculaires, Vols 1–4. Maîtres et Clefs de la Posture, Frères, Mairlot

Dart R 1950 Voluntary musculature in the human body: the double-spiral arrangement. British Journal of Physical Medicine 13(12NS):265–268

Edelman G 1992 Bright air, brilliant fire. Penguin, London

Godelieve D-S 1995 Le manuel du mezieriste. Editions Frison-Roche, Paris

Goldstein J 1999 Emergence as a construct: history and issues. Emergence: Complexity and Organization 1:49–72

Goodwin B 1994 How the leopard changed its spots. Phoenix, London

Gracovetsky S 1988 The spinal engine. Springer-Verlag, New York

Holland J 1998 Emergence – from chaos to order. Oxford University Press, Oxford

Jensen MC, Brant-Zawadzki MN, Obuchowski N et al 1994 Magnetic resonance imaging of the lumbar spine in people without back pain. New England Journal of Medicine 331(2):69–73

Johnson S 2001 Emergence – the connected lives of ants, brains, cities and software. Allen Lane, The Penguin Press, London

Kahneman D 2008 The third culture. (A talk by Daniel Kahneman) Edge 262: 22 October 2008. Online. Available: www.edge.org

Lakoff G, Johnson M 1980 Metaphors we live by. University of Chicago Press, Chicago

Long J 1995 The rise of fishes. University of New South Wales Press, Sydney

Mackenzie D 2008 Why the financial system is like an ecosystem. New Scientist 22 October 2008, 200(2679):8–9

McKenzie C, James K 2004 Aesthetics as an aid to understanding complex systems and decision judgement in operating complex systems. Emergence: Complexity and Organization 6(1,2):32–39

Morgan M, Morrison M 1999 Models as mediators. Cambridge University Press, Cambridge

Myers T 2009 Anatomy trains: myofascial meridians for manual and movement therapists, 2nd edn. Churchill Livingstone, Edinburgh

NASA Astrobiology Institute. Could life be based on silicon rather than carbon? http://nai.arc.nasa.gov/astrobio/feat_questions/silicon_life.cfm

Needham J 1936 Order and life. The M.I.T. Press, Cambridge, Massachusetts, p 108

Needham J et al 1954– Science and civilisation in China, 7 vols, ongoing. Cambridge University Press, Cambridge

O'Connor J, McDermott I 1997 The art of the systems thinking. Thorsons, London

O'Rahilly R, Müller F 1996 Human embryology & teratology, 2nd edn. Wiley-Liss, New York

Taylor W, Smeets L, Hall J, McPherson K 2004 The burden of rheumatic disorders in general practice: consultation rates for rheumatic disease and the relationship to age, ethnicity, and small-area deprivation. The New Zealand Medical Journal 117(1203)

Winchester S 2008 Bomb, book & compass; Joseph Needham and the great secrets of China. Penguin Viking, London

Lateral contractile field (L-CF) 4

The default movement pattern vertebrates have employed is a side-to-side undulation. This inherited pattern of movement is still the core curriculum for human locomotion.

Side-bending (also called lateral flexion; I use both terms interchangeably) of the torso is a core movement pattern that we have inherited from our piscean ancestors. The lateral contractile field (L-CF) is envisaged as a bilaminar ring of contractility that generously covers the lateral border of the head and torso. The term bilaminar refers to the external two layers of the trilaminar body-wall as the deep layer is modelled as contributing to the radial CF. The lateral eye and otic region of the sensory platform are embedded in the L-CF. To isolate the sensory platform from left/right swings of the torso, the field is modelled as crossing in the suboccipital region to the contralateral side of the neck. Here it then courses caudally along the lateral neck and torso to insert on the iliac crest of the pelvis. The lateral contractility then emerges as the remnants of our tail-wagging muscles, to then twist and cross the midline again via the perineal body of the pelvic floor. Thus, the field looks like a figure of eight with the ear and eye embedded in the upper ring. Side-bending is a powerful movement pattern that is a primal contributor to our ability to walk and run (Gracovetsky 1988).

67

DOI: 10.1016/B978-0-7020-3109-0.00009-2

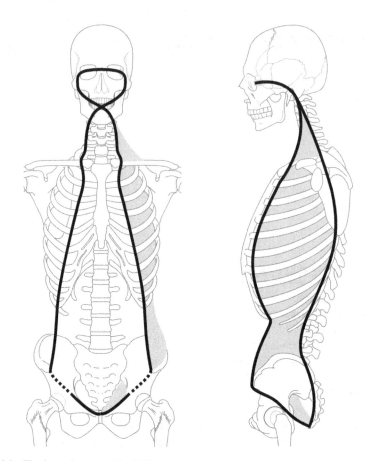

FIG 4.1 **The lateral contractile field** *Adapted from Beach 2007.*

EVOLUTIONARY PERSPECTIVE

Fish have had half a billion years to explore lateral contraction of the body-wall for swimming. From an evolutionary perspective, all vertebrates coalesce about two primary post-cranial muscle domains: the epimere that forms the dorsal muscle groups, and the hypomere that forms the lateral and ventral muscle groups. Each spinal nerve bifurcates into a primary dorsal and ventral nerve root, with the dorsal nerve supplying the muscles of the epimere, and the ventral nerve supplying the hypomere. The L-CF is derived from the hypomere of the vertebrate lateral body-wall and is innervated by the ventral rami.

The vast majority of fish species have developed a specialized mechanoreceptive sensory system that is attuned to water flow disturbances and low frequency sound waves. Early fish liberally distributed these sense organs (called neuromasts) over the lateral head and trunk but with time, they came to be collected and canalized into what is known as a lateral line system. The lateral line of jawed fish is often distinctly canalized as

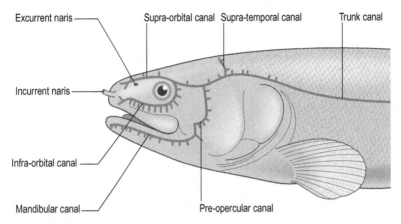

Excurrent naris — | Supra-orbital canal | Supra-temporal canal | Trunk canal
Incurrent naris —
Infra-orbital canal —
Mandibular canal —
Pre-opercular canal

FIG 4.2 **Distribution of the lateral line canals on the head of the bowfin, *Amia*** *Adapted from Liem et al Functional anatomy of the vertebrates, 3rd edn.© 2001 Brookes/Cole, a part of Cengage Learning, Inc. Reproduced by permission.*

the supraorbital, the infraorbital, and the mandibular canals, to then meander down the lateral flank of the fish body as a longitudinal pit(s) embedded with hair-like sense organs that monitor current dynamics. Even if a fish is blinded the lateral line is able to sense rocks and other fish so it is sometimes referred to as a receptor for distant touch. The lateral line develops from five or six neurogenic placodes that form in front of, and behind, the otic organ. A terrestrial existence did not need this type of sense organ. Biologists have long speculated that the lateral line sensory field was appropriated and became coiled up to contribute to a tetrapod's balance organs, the semi-circular canals of the inner ear (Liem et al 2001). The L-CF is modelled as having the otic region embedded within it, as this sensory region has always been associated with the lateral aspect of the vertebrate body-wall.

Moving from the aquatic environment to the terrestrial environment moved the onus for propulsion from the body-wall to the newly acquired limbs, but side-bending of the torso is still a core component of terrestrial gait patterning. Bipedalism placed additional new challenges on a well-evolved tetrapod gait pattern, specifically how to torque convert a side-bending of the spine to a rotary drive of the pelvis. To facilitate this torque conversion our iliac crest moved from a lateral orientation to a more ventral orientation, thus we have an *anterior* superior iliac spine (Aiello & Dean 1990). Now lateral flexion is usually coupled with a twisting forward or backward of the pelvis relative to the shoulders.

EMBRYOLOGICAL PERSPECTIVE

Mesoderm migrates from the dorsal body toward the ventral body with lateral folding of the embryonic disc. During this process mammals laminate the lateral musculature into three layers producing a trilaminar body-wall.

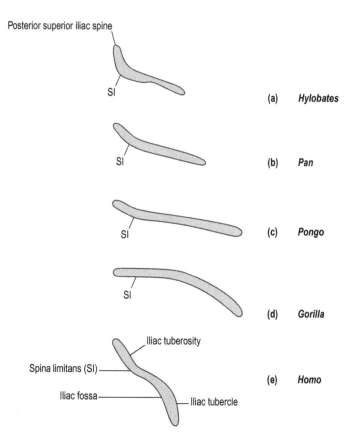

Posterior superior iliac spine

SI   (a)   *Hylobates*

SI   (b)   *Pan*

SI   (c)   *Pongo*

SI   (d)   *Gorilla*

Iliac tuberosity

Spina limitans (SI)

Iliac fossa

Iliac tubercle

(e)   *Homo*

FIG 4.3 Looking down on the top of the iliac crest of (a) gibbon, (b) chimpanzee, (c) orangutan, (d) gorilla, and (e) modern human Note the anterior swing of the human iliac crest. *Adapted from Aiello & Dean 1990.*

The external layer is obliquely angled downward and forward, and the internal oblique layer is obliquely directed downward and laterally, with the deepest layer roughly transverse. Migrating muscle cells must become influenced by morphogenetic fields that exert a strong diagonal pull that instils muscle fiber direction in the muscle layers. With further ventral migration the muscle precursor cells enter a presumed ventral field where they pinch away from the trilaminar body-wall and assume a longitudinal fiber orientation (here called the ventral domain of the dorso/ventro contractile field (D/V-CF)).

A nodal point within this field is the otic region. The lateral body-wall and the otic complex have co-evolved since the dawn of the vertebrate phyla. The ears, like the nose and eyes, first manifest as placodes that will invaginate to form the inner ear. The external ear, called the pinna, found only in mammals, forms from six hillocks of tissue that develop on the first and second pharyngeal arches. The hillocks coalesce and are concurrently drawn up and back toward the invaginating inner ear.

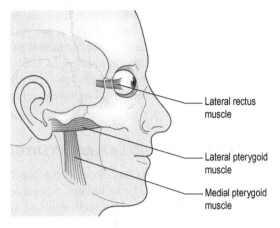

Lateral rectus muscle

Lateral pterygoid muscle

Medial pterygoid muscle

FIG 4.4   The lateral contractile field of the head region

FIELD DESCRIPTION

LATERAL RECTUS OF THE EYE

The external eye muscles have had a long but remarkably stable evolutionary history where six muscles seem to be the preferred, probably minimum, number of muscles to control a vertebrate's eyeball in its socket. The cranial nerves that power those six muscles are also deeply conserved. The sole function of cranial nerve VI (abducens) is the innervation of the lateral rectus, a small extrinsic muscle that pulls the eyeball laterally. For hundreds of millions of years lateral pulls to the vertebrate eyeball have had a dedicated cranial nerve, probably so that the eyeball can counter the propulsive lateral flexion of the caudal body. As fish do not have a neck, when they swim the head would tend to move left/right, making it difficult to visually track prey and move coherently. So the lateral rectus acting with the medial rectus decouples the eyes from the neck/torso and demonstrates the long association our body-plan has had with propulsion derived from bending side to side. If this muscle or nerve is compromised one develops double vision.

Another key aspect to modelling CFs are the righting reactions that are a crucial part of childhood development. When a baby is held up horizontally it will initially flop down. The head soon lifts to a more horizontal position in an attempt to right itself via the lateral rectus, the sternocleidomastoid/trapezius, and the lateral suboccipital muscles playing a role in the righting reaction. This is one of various righting reactions that are described, all of which are essential for the baby to progress in its development toward sitting and standing (Flehmig 1992). Because childhood righting reactions are so important to our normal development they have to be considered in each CF.

Most vertebrates place the orbits more to the side of the head. Humans, to facilitate binocular vision, bring the orbits frontally. Other animals that have orbits on the front of the face tend to be carnivores as vision becomes more focused for pinpointing targets and distance. The roof of the human orbit has developed a close relationship with the floor of the cranial cavity as our large frontal brain has pushed out over the top of the eyes. So at first glance the L-CF would seem to pass over the ears and up to the vertex of the head, but I suggest crossing the sensory platform via the lateral movement of the eyeball is a more cogent path to link the left and right L-CF. Two thousand years ago the Chinese came to a similar conclusion with the Gall Bladder meridian that zigzags up the lateral body-wall to the ear region to then cross to the lateral eye.

JAW MUSCLES – THE MEDIAL AND LATERAL PTERYGOID

A highly specialized group of muscles has developed to open and close the jaw. The most primitive chordates did not have a moveable jaw but, over time, a splendid array of vertebrate jaws and teeth evolved, with the temporomandibular joint (TMJ) being a mammalian innovation. Being warm-blooded and active requires a considerable food intake so mammals developed a jaw with specialized teeth that occluded tightly. To speed up digestion, food was pre-processed in the mouth by jaws that had developed a shearing and crushing capability, unlike the simple puncturing action of the reptilian jaw.

All the jaw muscles migrate to the region from the first pharyngeal arch. Here we need to introduce more embryology. Along the length of the embryo the somites manifest. From the somites the vertebrae and muscles associated with each somite will emerge, with some of the muscles migrating a considerable distance from the somite of origin. In the region of the head, overt somites do not appear, but seven pre-somitic whorls of mesodermal tissue can be seen with a scanning electron microscope – the whorls are called somitomeres. The first, second, third, and fifth somitomeres are thought to contribute to the extrinsic six muscles of the eyeball. These muscles represent the apex of the neuromuscular system.

The fourth somitomere contributes the precursor mesoderm that will migrate to the first pharyngeal arch to form the jaw muscles, all innervated by the trigeminal nerve (V), the nerve of the first pharyngeal arch (Liem et al 2001). These muscles are the temporalis, the masseter, and the medial and lateral pterygoid, with another couple of small muscles that act on the ear. All of these muscles are placed on the lateral jaw and temple, so all could be considered as being embedded in the L-CF. However, the medial and lateral pterygoid, due to their crossed form, deep location, and their ability to deviate the mandible laterally, suggest to me the way to model these complex muscles is to place the pterygoids as the cardinal muscles of the L-CF in the jaw region.

OTIC REGION

The ear itself, the auricularis muscles that act on the pinna, the stylohyoid, the posterior belly of the digastric, and the small muscles of the inner ear are modelled as being embedded in the L-CF.

TONGUE

The anterior portion of the tongue is formed by a fusion of left and right moieties, with a single midline development contributing to the root of the tongue. Thus the tongue is modelled as being a fusion of the ventral domain of the D/V-CF (the root of the tongue) and the L-CF (the sides of the tongue).

STERNOCLEIDOMASTOID (SCM) AND TRAPEZIUS

Both of these muscles are derived from a muscle called the cucullaris, which lifted the gills of fish (Wake 1979). A terrestrial existence made gills obsolete but the cucullaris adapted by migrating to the skull and pectoral girdle on the dorsal body and the sternum/clavicles of the ventral body. Because of this shared evolutionary origin, some anatomists see the two muscles as a complex single muscle that has split apart.

The SCM and the trapezius share a common innervation by a cranial nerve, the accessory nerve (XI). The nerve arises from a series of rootlets that originate both rostral to, and between the dorsal and ventral roots of the spinal nerves C1–C5/6. The rootlets form a trunk that enters the foramen magnum, to emerge back through the skull via the jugular foramen. So, although the nerve is termed a cranial nerve, the spinal component that interests us here is derived from the cervical spine.

The SCM is one of the most unusual muscles of the body in that it is able to intervene in many movement patterns. Acting together, the SCM and trapezius are able to side-bend the head on the neck so that, for example, if the torso side-bends left the head is able to side-bend right. De-coupling the head from the torso and lower cervical spine is essential to all of our movement patterns.

RECTUS CAPITIS LATERALIS, SUPERIOR OBLIQUE, AND SPLENIUS CAPITUS

These are small muscles that side-bend the occiput on the upper neck. They act with the SCM and trapezius to contralateral side-bend the head on the neck during righting reactions.

MIDDLE SCALENE, INTERCOSTALS INTERNI, INTERNAL OBLIQUE; POSTERIOR SCALENE, INTERCOSTALS EXTERNI, EXTERNAL OBLIQUE

Here we have six named muscles that are all derived from a similar embryonic layer. As explained earlier, the posterior scalene, the intercostals externi, and the external oblique form a continuous layer of muscle from the iliac crest to the suboccipital region of the neck. Likewise, the middle scalene, the intercostals interni, and the internal oblique form a deeper layer with muscle fiber direction roughly at right angles to the external layer. A key insight in the modelling of this CF was to separate the external two layers named above from the deepest muscle layer of our trilaminar body-wall. I attribute the inner layer of the trilaminar body-wall to the radial contractile field (R-CF).

The vertebrate body-plan has a distinct ventral and dorsal midline. In contrast the lateral body-wall does not exhibit a distinct border between ventral and dorsal. If you look at someone from the side, where does the dorsal body meet the ventral body? It is a border region rather than a strict demarcation. The external and internal obliques control this regional border by generously covering it in contractile tissues that pull in obliquely opposite directions. If both muscles pull equally the body will 'pure' side-bend. Most of the time the body will side-bend with an element of flexion or extension as one of the obliques becomes dominant. Control of the lateral body-wall is thus inherently unstable with side-bending usually coupled with flexion or extension of the torso.

The L-CF forms a boundary with the dorsal domain of the D/V-CF at the rib angles on the dorsal body-wall. It is as though the ribs push their bone through the muscle layers to create a distinct dorsal/lateral regionalization. The field is bounded in the lumbar region by the lateral raphe (a fascial condensation) that marks the lateral junction of the caudal erector spinae muscles with the abdominal wall muscle. Ventrally the L-CF borders the ventral domain of the D/V-CF at the rib costo-chondral junction of the rib cage, and the linea semilunaris of the abdominal wall, to then insert along the iliac crest.

Two layers of muscle cloak the lateral body-wall of the torso. The L-CF is wide and powerful in the mid-chest region, repeatedly braced and strengthened by the ribs. Lateral musculature cones down as it approaches the top ribs, then continues as the posterior and middle scalene to the lateral margins of C2–C7. Hence a massive side-bending force is brought to bear on the lateral margins of the lower six cervical vertebrae. Note how this arrangement allows the head to de-couple from the neck/torso via the contralateral SCM/trapezius complex.

At the caudal end of the body, the external and internal oblique insert on the iliac crest from the lateral raphe posterially to the anterior superior iliac spine (ASIS). Again the two muscle layers are repeated braced by the ribs in a wide area of origin from the rib angles to the costo-chondral junction. A broad multisegmental force is focused on the relatively small iliac crest so that contractility is wide and slow over the lateral region of the middle ribs (useful as hearts, lungs, stomach, and liver reside internally and probably need some isolation from explosive contractility) but short and powerful in their action on the pelvis.

COCCYGEUS, ILIOCOCCYGEUS, AND PERINEAL BODY OF THE PELVIC FLOOR

Following the ilia caudally, the field re-emerges as contractile tissue that will laterally tail-wag the sacrum and coccyx (the ischiococcygeus and iliococcygeus). As we will see when we discuss the D/V-CF, the pelvic floor is a melee of muscular/fascial directional interchange with the perineal body as a nodal region. Conceptually, I suggest the left and right lateral fields twist across the caudal pole of the body that external musculature on the right becomes continuous with a deeper, internal fascial plane on the left, and vice versa.

Imagine a ribbon with diagonal lines of opposite orientation drawn on the two sides. If the two ends of the ribbon are joined to make a circle the diagonal lines stay separate. If, however, the ribbon is pinched and twisted 180 degrees the internal diagonal becomes the external diagonal on the contralateral side. I suspect this is what happens in the embryological development of these muscles. A single sheet of contractility is impressed with fiber orientation on

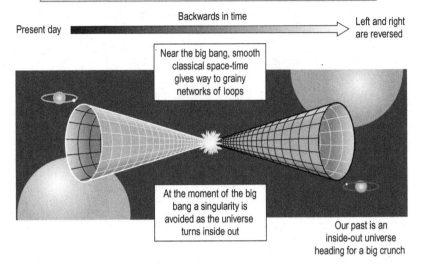

FIG 4.5 **A diagram from *New Scientist* depicting a new model of the 'big bang', used here to model the decussation of the lateral fields** The outside twists become the inside so the internal oblique on one side is the external oblique on the contralateral side. *Adapted from Gefter 2004.*

both sides, it twists at the perineal body, and then laminates into two sheets. Above is a diagram from a *New Scientist* article that discussed a new theory of the 'big bang' called Loop Quantum Cosmology (Gefter 2004). Depicting the origin of the universe as similar to the unity of the two sides of the L-CF is somewhat speculative!

REFERENCES

Aiello L, Dean C 1990 An introduction to human evolutionary anatomy. Academic Press, London

Beach P 2007 The contractile field – a new model of human movement, Part 1. Journal of Bodywork and Movement Therapies 11(4):308–317

Flehmig I 1992 Normal infant development and borderline deviations. Thieme, New York

Gefter A 2004 The world turned inside out. Was the big bang the start of everything? New Scientist 181(2439):34

Gracovetsky S 1988 The spinal engine. Springer-Verlag Wein, New York

Liem K, Bemis W, Walker W, Grande L 2001 Functional anatomy of the vertebrates, 3rd edn. Harcourt, Fort Worth

Wake M 1979 Hyman's comparative vertebrate anatomy, 3rd edn. University of Chicago Press, Chicago

Dorso/ventro contractile field (D/V-CF)

5

A terrestrial existence challenged vertebrate locomotor design. The spinal complex
responded to gravity and friction by developing regional complexity and exploring new planes
of movement. Spinal flexion and extension became important to how tetrapods move.

This field manifests as rings of bilateral, para-axial contractile tissue. The
rings cross and fuse as they encircle the dorsal and ventral length of the body.
Of particular interest are the regions where the dorsal and ventral domains
meet, and where they cross the midline to left/right meld, which the contractility surely must. Dividing the dorso/ventro contractile field (D/V-CF) into
dorsal and ventral domains is useful for analysis. However, when considering a whole-organism approach to movement it is the relationship between
the domains that is the interesting part. As the Chinese say of their midline
meridians:

> *The Conception and Governing vessels are like midday and midnight, they are the*
> *polar axis of the body ... there is one source and two branches, one goes to the front*
> *and the other goes to the back of the body ... When we try to divide these, we see*
> *that yin and yang are inseparable. When we try to see them as one, we see that it is*
> *an indivisible whole.*

Maciocia 1998, p. 496

The interplay of the lateral contractile field (L-CF) and the D/V-CF are very
tightly coupled to manage the shape of the body, as movement is the coherent

© 2010 Elsevier Ltd / Inc / Bv
DOI: 10.1016/B978-0-7020-3109-0.00010-9

changing of shape. As a thought experiment, imagine a tube of thick plasticine shaped like the torso. If the left and right L-CF were to both contract, the plasticine would shorten and protrude front and back to produce a hunch back with a potbelly. The D/V-CF would immediately kick in to limit this type of shape deformation. Likewise, if both the dorsal and the ventral domains of the D/V-CF were to contract, the plasticine would again shorten, but this time plasticine would protrude in the lateral direction like a severe scoliosis. Again, this would elicit a shape-managing reflex that would see the L-CF contracting to limit the lateral deformation. The vertebrate torso has a spinal system that strongly resists this type of simplistic shape change but the thought experiment is useful in demonstrating how deeply shape coupled these two CFs are. From this perspective the L-CF and the D/V-CF are similar to the agonist/antagonist relations between individual muscles. In Chapter 6, I will show how the lumbar spine has created a form of spinal gearbox from this coupling.

EVOLUTIONARY PERSPECTIVE

The dorsal domain of the field is derived from the epaxial musculature of fish and is similarly innervated by the dorsal rami of the spinal nerves. The ventral domain of this D/V-CF is derived from the ventral edge of the hypomere of fish (the lateral plate of embryology); nerve supply is via ventral rami of the spinal nerves. At the neck/head region this field is continuous with the hypobranchial muscles that migrate up to the tongue region, ventral to the gills or pharyngeal arches. Tongues have a rich evolutionary history as they became mobile and associated with many primary functions such as food acquisition and manipulation, swallowing, taste, teeth, and speech.

A terrestrial life facilitated the exploration of flexion/extension movements as the spinal column became more complexly regionalized and jointed. Spinal extensor muscles lift the head on the neck for feeding, extend spinal segments locally and regionally, and lift the tail when alert or defecating.

EMBRYOLOGICAL PERSPECTIVE

Briefly recapping: before longitudinal 'folding' of the embryo (day 22), the anterior pole of the embryonic disc contains the precursive cardiogenic cells and the septum transversum. The caudal pole of the embryonic disc hosts precursive mesoderm that will contribute to the future lower abdominal wall. Folding brings those polar structures to meet in the region of the navel and the lower abdomen.

At the same time the embryo is folding laterally. Mesoderm follows this folding to migrate first laterally and then ventrally to eventually meet at the ventral midline. Precursive muscle tissue, as it migrates ventrally, enters a para-midline morphogenetic field that mandates a change in fiber direction to become cephalically/caudally orientated, as seen in the rectus abdominis.

The primitive streak and the ensuing notochord confer a strict left/right division to the embryonic disc. Mesoderm that finds itself left stays left, and vice versa. However, a pinching together of the epiblast to the endoblast halts the cephalic and caudal midline development of the notochord. The cephalic pinching is called the buccopharyngeal membrane; it will perforate later on to be the future mouth. The caudal midline pinching is called the cloacal membrane; it will later breakdown to form the anal and genitourinary orifices (see Fig. 2.6).

Above and below these two tightly pinched areas, the laterally migrating mesoderm is able to cross the midline. Mesodermal migration across the region cephalic to the buccopharyngeal membrane will be important to the formation of the ventral chest wall and diaphragm; in the pelvic floor region it allows mesoderm to interpenetrate across the midline. Your dorsal body-wall musculature is strictly left/right divided whereas parts of your ventral body-wall are a profound interweaving of left and right mesodermal tissue.

THE DORSAL DOMAIN OF THE DORSO/VENTRO-CF

OLFACTORY REGION

Imagine you are sitting Japanese style on the floor as I reach over your head to use two of my fingers to pull you backward, trying to extend your head on your neck. If my contact point were the superior/medial margin of your orbits you would feel unable to resist as your delicate lacrimal bones risk collapse, with very unpleasant complications. Likewise, if I gripped your nostrils with my index and middle finger and pulled backward the result is predictable. No matter how strong your abdominal wall and neck flexors are I would be able to pull you into extension. Sense organs are just too biologically important, fragile, and valuable to risk. I have you by a control point. All systems have control points. If you want to influence a system, knowledge of the network of control is essential.

Let us try another gripped image. This time I use my fingers to grip you between the upper teeth and the top lip – the labial sulcus. Again, you will extend. Following on, this time I grip your upper four middle teeth (the incisors) and pull you backward – this time I am the one in trouble, big trouble. By moving my grip less than an inch I have gone from being the controller to being the badly bitten. All the considerable power of your jaw and neck/abdo flexors is now unleashed for your resistance. Not only that, because fingers are important to a primate, you now command. A field threshold has been crossed.

The nose is a sense organ of the central nervous system (CNS) – the CNS of vertebrates is by definition a dorsal body structure. The vertebrate body-plan features an embryonic forebrain called the telencephalon from which the olfactory sense is derived – it is a deeply conserved relationship. All vertebrates place the nose at or near the anterior leading edge of the animal, as it has to be near the mouth for odor sampling. The dorsal body meets the ventral body at the junction of the nose and the teeth.

The first embryonic hint of a nose on the massive 'head' (which at this early stage is all brain pushing out from its dural fascial tethering) is two nasal embryonic placodes. They appear during the fourth week, facing

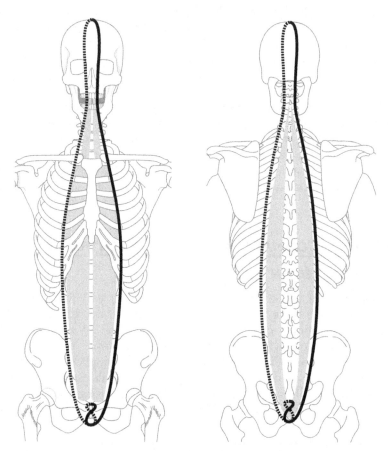

FIG 5.1 *Dorsal domain* **of the D/V-CF** Modelled as including the nose, superior/inferior rectus of the eye, occipito-frontalis, the erector spinae, pubo-coccygeal, the infra-umbilical portion of the rectus abdominis. *Ventral domain* Including the incisors, temporalis/ masseter, the root of the tongue, midline supra/infra hyoid muscles, the SCM with the anterior vertebral neck flexors, the parasternal interchondral complex, rectus abdominis to the infra-umbilical region. *Adapted from Beach 2007.*

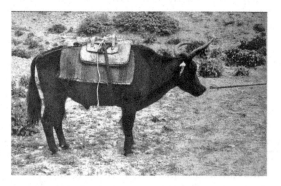

FIG 5.2 **Led by the nose: a Tibetan dzo, half yak and half cow, a huge animal** Just outside the photograph a 12-year-old girl is able to control this animal via an attachment to a critical point in the animal's morphology.

anterio/laterally. The placodes invaginate toward the underlying brain and medial and lateral nasal processes emerge. As the embryo matures about the ventral midline the two 'noses' meet and fuse to produce the recognizable nose.

The dorsal domain covers the width of the nose, the maxillary labial vestibule, and above, the superior/medial area of the orbit. Conceptually the left and right nasal fields will narrow and fuse at the bridge of the nose, to then twist. Olfactory nerves (cranial I) pass directly backward to the olfactory bulb of the brain without intermediate neurons, with the left olfactory nerve linking predominantly with the left brain and the right olfactory nerve linking predominantly to the right brain. Therefore, the left nose links to the left brain but by the time we get to the left erector spinae muscles the right brain is in charge. A form of neurological decussation has taken place.

If your head is pulled into extension, initially you will look up (superior rectus), but again a threshold is reached and you look down as part of a righting reaction (going too far backward is biomechanical bad news so your system initiates a protective righting reaction). With extension of the head your jaw tends to open, the nasal orifices tend to dilate (dilatator naris) and the occipito-frontalis will corrugate your forehead.

ERECTOR SPINAE

To lift a bodily region relative to the whole organism a stable region is needed from which to act. The thoracic organs need to maintain their intra-compartmental space for functionality. For example, the heart is an organ that needs a substantially braced compartment that will contain, dampen, and protectively isolate its pulsatile movement. The first to fifth thoracic vertebrae and ribs are amongst the first wave of bones to manifest and ossify. The upper thorax is well braced dorsally and ventrally to act as a stable region for flexing/extending the head/neck on the thorax, and likewise the sacrum/caudal region extends via muscle fibers that originate in the upper thoracic region. So within the D/V-CF the upper thoracic spinal region is relatively stable and braced.

Developmentally and neurologically, it makes sense to view the erector spinae as a cascade of musculature, from cephalic to caudal. Long columns of muscle run down your back, all innervated via the dorsal ramus of the spinal nerves. The erector spinae have been extensively studied. The following classification system (Bogduk 1997) is a useful way to make sense of this complicated mass of muscle fibers.

Unisegmental muscles (interspinales, intertransversarii)

These muscles cross from one vertebral segment to the next below. They are small and close to the action pivot so they cannot exert a large movement force on a segment, but they are packed with sensory nerve endings that monitor segmental dynamics. Also they have a protective function. When a load threatens to take a segment into the distress zone these small muscles clamp tightly together to protect their segmental level, each segment passing the abhorrent load along until a 'fall guy' segment is load damaged.

Polysegmental muscles (multifidus)

These are muscles that cross over the segment immediately below to insert 2/3/4/5 segments caudally. Every vertebral segment has thousands of muscle fibers originating at that level. Those muscles all pass caudally, and are innervated by the spinal nerve that issues from the segment of origin. Thus each spinal segment is in control of a muscular army that all originate on that segment, linking to many segments caudally.

Long polysegmental muscles (longissimus and iliocostalis)

These muscles link a spinal segment to distal segments, terminating on the dorsal iliac crest and the dorsal surface of the sacrum.

No erector spinae originates lateral to your rib angles so this bony feature marks the lateral border of this field. It is as if the ribs' angles have, in part, pushed themselves through the external body-wall musculature to largely separate the L-CF from the dorsal domain of the D/V-CF (note that the L-CF will send some contractile tissue deep to the erector spinae, to be expected as CFs meld to a structural/functional whole). Below the ribs the lateral limit of the field is the lateral raphe. The lateral raphe is a fascial condensation formed where the abdominal muscles meet the lateral lumbar erector spinae.

Fascial depth change is expected in the CF model, just as textiles must warp and weft. The trapezius is the only muscle to lie superficial to the erector spinae as they insert onto the occiput. The relatively superficial erector spinae complex then dives deeper in the facial layers to again re-emerge in the T6/T7/T8 region. Again the erector starts to dive deep to pass under and through the thoracolumbar fascia. The anatomy of this fascia is complex but some of it is derived from the abdominal muscles. In the thoracic region the abdominal muscles are represented by the intercostals, which the erector group is superficial to. So when the erector spinae dive under and through the thoracolumbar fascia they now pass deep to some of the abdominal fascia, hence another depth change. As the erector emerges to insert on the sacrum it is again a superficial muscle.

As muscle rises and falls within the fascial envelope of the body it also narrows and widens. The dorsal field narrows as it inserts on the base of the skull. As we descend the dorsal field it widens to a maximum at rib 6/7/8/9, then begins to cone down toward an insertion area on the dorsal surface of the sacrum (and the iliac tuberosity of the iliac crest). Again, we have muscle from many segments (as far away as T4/T5) which, when the bony surface area is combined, offers a large area for attachment (neural arches, transverse processes, ribs as far laterally as the rib angle), thus focusing multi-segmental power on a narrowed caudal spinal region. If you have to, you can move your head and tail quickly and forcefully. In my osteopathic practice I see so many more cases of pulled low back muscles compared with upper back muscles that I suspect this is designed into the system. Like the front of a car that is designed to crush on impact, the low back is meant to strain rather than the thoracic origin of the muscle. A strain in the thoracic region can make it hard to breathe; compared with breathing with pain, walking with pain is a minor irritation.

Pelvic floor – pubococcygeal muscle

The sacrum is not the caudal terminus of the dorsal domain of the D/V-CF. Embryological folding takes caudal mesoderm from the sacral region to the ventral body, contributing to the musculature of the pelvic floor, the genitalia, and the abdominal wall overlying the bladder. If caudal folding is obstructed the baby may be born with an exposed bladder. So, in a deep sense the lower abdominal wall is derived from dorsal/extensor muscle. To visualize the functional importance of this muscular migration, imagine a patient lying prone and you want to lift his or her pelvis. Place your forearm on the patient's back and grip the skin over the sacrum, then try to lift up the sacrum and pelvis. It does not really work – you will just pull skin and hurt the patient. Likewise, a pull of the erector spinae will exert a compressive force on the lumbo-sacral region with only a small extension vector. However, if you carefully reach between the patient's legs and place your fingers on the lower abdomen and then pull up you will lift their caudal body into extension. Dorsal erector spinae muscles extend your body because of this ventral migration of their sphere of contractile activity.

Consider how the sacrum cones down to the bony terminus at the tip of the tail-like coccygeal vertebrae (which, during the early stages of embryogenesis, are described as being slightly spiralized off to one side). As a result of this coning down toward the coccygeal tip, left and right mean less and less, meeting then at the midline. Immediately post-tail is the anus, which is characterized by interlacing rings of contractile tissues (external anal sphincter) that are under voluntary nervous control. Moving further ventrally is the perineal body, a pyramidal fibromuscular node that nine muscles fuse with. This structure is morphologically complex. Muscles converge at the perineal body from different planes, spiralize, reform into bundles, and re-merge. The perineal body is essential for faecal and urinary continence. The migration of the early pioneer muscle cells that are pulled ventrally during folding cross the midline to contribute to the muscles that form around the pelvic orifices. In this way, the right and left erector spinae are twisted together to contribute to the contractility that forms the external muscular rings of the anal and urogenital orifices.

Taken as a whole, the muscle that carries on from the erector spinae to the pubis via the perineal body is called the pubococcygeal muscle, a portion of the pelvic floor muscle, the levator ani. The pubococcygeal muscle is the muscle that brings a dog's tail between its legs. As we lost our mobile tail the muscle was recruited to help form a more substantial pelvic floor that was required to cope with the new gravitational and intra-abdominal pressures that bipedalism placed on the pelvis, compounded by birthing issues required for our large-brained babies.

CFs are expected to cross the midline when possible, they are expected to rise and fall through fascial layers, and they are expected to widen and narrow like a river. The dorsal domain of the D/V-CF does just this on its journey from the olfactory region as it has changed fascial depth, widened and narrowed, and twisted to continue toward the navel as the caudal portion of the rectus abdominis.

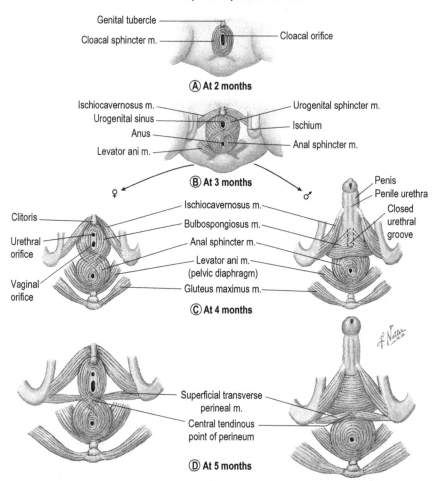

Prenatal development of perineal musculature

Genital tubercle

Cloacal sphincter m. — Cloacal orifice

(A) At 2 months

Ischiocavernosus m. — Urogenital sphincter m.
Urogenital sinus — Ischium
Anus — Anal sphincter m.
Levator ani m.

(B) At 3 months

♀   ♂

Clitoris — Ischiocavernosus m. — Penis / Penile urethra / Closed urethral groove
Urethral orifice — Bulbospongiosus m.
 — Anal sphincter m.
Vaginal orifice — Levator ani m. (pelvic diaphragm)
 — Gluteus maximus m.

(C) At 4 months

Superficial transverse perineal m.
Central tendinous point of perineum

(D) At 5 months

FIG 5.3 When the caudal body of the embryo folds, the precursive muscle tissue is drawn into a morphogenic field that flows around the cloacal region and on to the lower abdomen. *Adapted from Cochard 2002; Netter Illustration Collection at www.netterimages.com, with permission.* © Elsevier Inc. All rights reserved.

THE VENTRAL DOMAIN OF THE DORSO/VENTRO-CF

RECTUS ABDOMINIS

Contractility has been drawn from the spinal region to the pubic region, twisting left and right on the way. A remnant of that twisting is found as the pubococcygeus blends with the caudal insertion of the rectus abdominis. The lateral fibers of the rectus abdominis insert on the ipsilateral crest of the pubis (as expected), whereas the more medial fibers cross, in part, to the contralateral pubic bone. In the bodybuilder in Figure 5.4, note how the caudal end of the left and right rectus appears to blend across the midline. Note that the

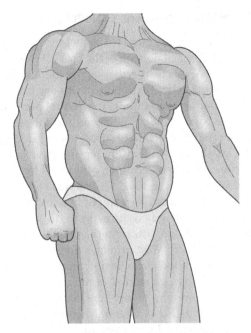

FIG 5.4 Tendinous intersections divide each rectus into usually three sections Each of the 'packs' draws on two or three ribs so that flexion is spread across segments. This arrangement allows a regionalized but braced control of abdominal flexion and extension.

caudal end of the rectus abdominis is a deep muscle as the transversus abdominis in this region has risen to cover the caudal rectus abdominis with its fascia.

The lateral edge of the rectus abdominis is called the linea-semilunaris because of its half-moon shape; it demarcates the lateral border of this field from the L-CF. The midline linea alba is a tendinous raphe formed from (white) fascial sheets derived from all the abdominal muscles. It has a small muscle (the pyramidalis that inserts on the pubis) that acts to tune and tether its functional tone.

The rectus abdominis is a ventral bilateral paraxial muscle that spans the pubis to the thorax. On many tetrapods this muscle extends high up the ribs; in humans it is attached to the fifth, sixth, and seventh costal cartilages. It is variable, sometimes extending as far rostrally as the third costal cartilage. Note how the rectus abdominis does not attach to the sternum. From this broad attachment the muscle descends with three (sometimes more) tendinous intersections that are in gym speak 'the six-pack.'

Each portion of the six-pack incorporates two rib segments. If each spinal segment did segment the rectus abdominis, as found in many lower terrestrial vertebrates, power generated by the muscle would be too local. A strong local contraction could pop a rib rather than move the torso. By bunching two rib segments together the rectus is able to trade between a nuanced flexion and the dissipation of force over multiple spinal segments.

PARASTERNAL INTERCHONDRAL COMPLEX

How does this field traverse the thorax? I model the linea semilunaris as the lateral border of the abdominal domain of the D/V-CF. Moving onto the chest wall, the lateral border of this field is marked by the costo-chondral junction (i.e. the joints between the ventral extremity of ribs one to seven and the costal cartilages, that then link rib to sternum). The ventral domain courses toward the neck between the costo-chondral junctions and the sternum.

The sternum is a complex bone that I suspect is an interloper in the ventral domain. Fish and snakes lack a sternum, reptiles have a U-shaped pectoral girdle, and birds have a massive sternum for the attachment of powerful wing muscles. Embryologically, two cartilaginous sternal bars emerge in the space between the ribs. They then fuse like a zipper in a rostral to caudal direction. Encircling ribs send out cartilaginous growths that join with the sternal bars. A variable number of bone growth centers emerge in the manubrium, the sternal body, and the xiphoid. Most primates do not fuse the sternum as we tend to, so their thorax will be more flexible than ours. Chimpanzees most closely approach our degree of sternal ossification (Aiello & Dean 1990). Pectoralis major, a limb muscle, inserts on the sternal bars, so in the CF context the sternum is modelled as a ventral component of the pectoral girdle just as the scapula is a lateral/dorsal element.

The ventral domain courses over and embeds the costal cartilages, and the muscles found between the costal cartilages – the parasternal interchondral muscles. These muscles need explaining. Ribs have three layers of intercostal muscles: the external, internal, and intimi. The external intercostal is red fiber from the rib area deep to the erector spinae to near the end of the ventral bony ribs, where it then turns into an external parasternal intercostal membrane. Conversely, the internal intercostal is red fiber from the interchondral region ventrally to the rib angle, where it turns into an internal intercostal membrane as it courses toward the dorsal midline. So the interchondral portion of the ribs is myostructurally different to the more lateral intercostal complex, and has a distinct innervation via the most ventral branches of the intercostal nerves.

THE THROAT AND JAW VIA THE MIDLINE INFRA AND SUPRA HYOID MUSCLES, THE STERNOCLEIDOMASTOID (SCM) WITH THE CERVICAL ANTERIOR VERTEBRAL MUSCLES, AND THE MASSETER/TEMPORALIS

Be prepared to re-read this a number of times because as contractility approaches the cranial region it takes on another order of complexity. In essence, the D/V-CF model has to address three imperatives here. Firstly, para-midline contractility must ascend to the lower jaw to flex the head on the neck, to depress the jaw, and to fuse across the midline at the tongue. Secondly, a bilateral para-midline contractility must be able to brace itself laterally, without which the head would be unstable when flexed. The SCM and the masseters/temporalis offer this lateral bracing. Thirdly, flexion of the head on the neck must be able to switch to extension of the head on the neck for those essential righting reactions.

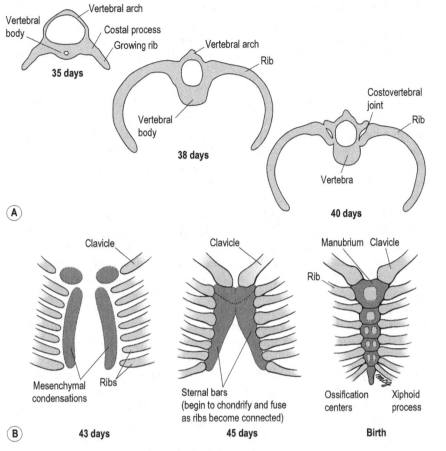

FIG 5.5 **The sternum is a complex and variable bone** The manubrium usually has one to three centers of ossification, whilst the two sternal bars fuse across the midline to form four units called sternebrae, each with one or two centers of ossification. If the sternum does not fuse, breathing is dramatically compromised. Note that the encircling ribs are derived from vertebral elements whereas the sternal bars are not. *Adapted from Schoenwolf et al 2008.*

The throat and jaw region are derived from the gill-like pharyngeal region of the embryo. During embryonic folding the large heart descends from the neck to the thorax whilst the CNS of the dorsal body ascends – the ascending and descending leaving a collapsed-looking neck (Blechschmidt & Gasser 1978). The ventral domain of the D/V-CF must emerge from this morass to, in a stable manner, flex the head on the neck, and the head/neck on the thorax. As flexion courses up from the low abdomen and the para-sternal region toward the neck/head I model the ventral domain as continuing to the root of the tongue via the para-midline infra and supra hyoid muscles. From an evolutionary perspective this group of muscles are called the hypo-branchials, as they lie ventral to the gill apparatus (Liem et al 2001). They migrate from the most caudal head segments and the anterior trunk segments toward the sternal region then up toward the tongue and jaw. They assist in opening the lower jaw and expanding the pharynx. Only muscles that insert or take off from the portion of the hyoid bone between the lesser cornu are modelled as being in the ventral domain of the D/V-CF. They include the sternohyoid, sternothyroid, thyrohyoid, geniohyoid, and the genioglossus. Within the ventral domain I embed the chin (only humans have chins), the incisors, and the root of the tongue.

Fish have a tongue-like structure called the primary tongue. It is not muscular and plays no role in the manipulation of food. The tongue of tetrapods has become a varied and versatile organ that is crucial to eating and swallowing, tasting and talking. In some bats the tongue extends back as far as the sternum (Kent 1992), whilst chameleons anchor the tongue as far back as the pelvis. Mammals use the tongue to place food between the upper and lower dentition. On the tongue are taste buds that bear a long evolutionary co-development with the olfactory sense.

Our tongue and the articulation it allows us play a pivotal role in all human evolutionary scenarios. Talking has literally created us. The tongue is an organ that has to be tough enough to move rough food quickly between hard tearing and grinding surfaces but must also command extraordinary delicacy in the control of airflow for our complex vocalization. So how does the tongue change its shape so fluently, in dangerous conditions, without cartilaginous or skeletal support?

Body support systems can be divided into two categories. The first category uses either hardened internal (endoskeleton) and/or external (exoskeletal) elements to facilitate movement. The second category is that of the non-rigid type, the hydroskeletons, as found in many of the early body-plans. The tongue (and octopus arms and the trunk of an elephant) fits somewhere between these two categories. It is a muscular hydrostat – an organ made entirely of muscle. There are three primary muscle fiber directions: longitudinal, transverse, and left/right helical. The tongue is incompressible so it is protruded and thin or retracted and fat. Helical fibers are essential to move the tongue around the lip vestibules by twisting the tongue along its long axis. But it still retains a midline septa and frenulum, and the terminal nerve supply is largely left/right separate, as evidenced by a unilateral section of the hypoglossal nerve yielding an ipsilateral limp and atrophy. Higher up the neurological command chain, the nuclei in the brain stem are left/right cross-wired so unilateral lesions here do not still the tongue as the contralateral nuclei can (to a degree) compensate.

Embryologically, the tongue arises from the floor of the pharynx. A fusion of three embryonic growth centers derived from the first branchial arch amalgamate to form the anterior two-thirds of the tongue. Mesoderm from the occipital somites (embryonic somites that extend rostral to the cervical somites) migrates ventrally into the tongue bud to form the intrinsic musculature of the tongue (the lingual muscle). The hypoglossal nerve (cranial XII) supplies motor innervation to the tongue. Cranial XII is found in series with the ventral rami of the spinal nerves; it can be seen as a cranial extension of the cervical spinal nerves that got trapped in the developing skull. I hypothesize that both evolutionary and developmental perspectives suggest the tongue represents a fusion of both lateral and ventral morphogenic fields. If that fusion does not occur, a forked tongue results, a common condition in reptiles, but thankfully reassuringly rare in mammals.

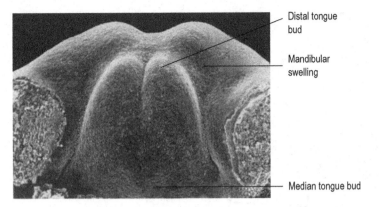

Distal tongue
bud

Mandibular
swelling

Median tongue bud

FIG 5.6 Embryonic tongue, early sixth week The lateral tongue buds (called 'distal' on the photograph) grow to become the anterior two-thirds of the tongue. There is a fusion of left/right and the ventral domain. *From Larsen 1993.*

We have now followed the ventral domain from the low abdomen to the root of the tongue. From a neuromuscular perspective we have ascended to the lingual muscles that are derived from occipital somites and innervated by cranial XII. If we continue to ascend the neuromuscular tree rostral to the tongue we must look to muscles that are innervated by cranial nerves above cranial XII. Contractility can ascend via the SCM (acting with the cervical anterior vertebral muscles) and the masseter/temporalis muscles and, in doing so, add a left/right stability to flexion of the head/neck complex. If the ventral domain was only para-midline, then flexion of the head on the neck would easily buckle the head on the neck. By modelling the ventral domain as both inserting into the tongue and coursing laterally to the sides of the head, the flexion is strong and stable. The SCM accessory nerve (cranial XI) acting bilaterally is an obvious head/neck flexor, but that is so only if it acts with the deep flexors of the cervical spine (the longus colli and the longus capitus).

Masseter and temporalis are muscles that are derived from the first pharyngeal arch, which is, by definition, a ventral structure. All the muscles derived from this arch are innervated by the trigeminal nerve (cranial V). Both muscles are very strong and both close the jaw. Flexion of the body and the head on the neck carry the ventral domain to meet with the dorsal domain of the D/V-CF, and via the SCM, contractility is carried to the lateral aspects of the skull where they meld in with the L-CF.

At an anatomically deep level, flexion and extension pivot at the sphenobasilar junction. In your 20s this joint fuses, thus locking in a fundamental relationship between flexion and extension.

The third imperative to be considered is the issue of a flexion of the head on the neck being able to switch easily to an extension of the head on the neck, that is, a tipping point that is essential to the righting reactions. A supine newborn, when pulled up to sit by the arms, will demonstrate almost complete head lag. At 2 months there is less head lag, and by 4 months there is no head lag. It takes an average of 4 months for the baby to develop the

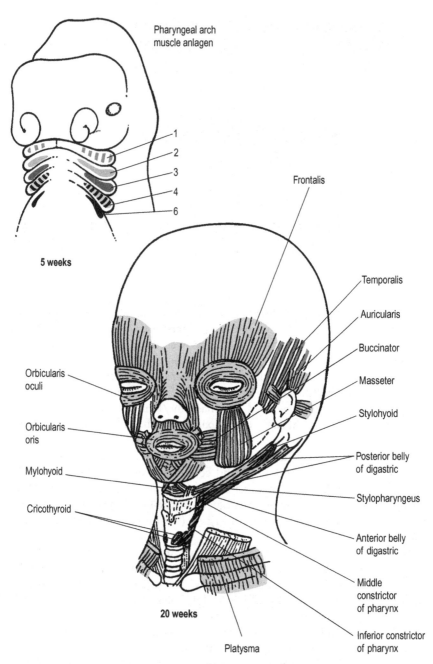

Pharyngeal arch
muscle anlagen

1
2
3
4
6

5 weeks

Frontalis

Temporalis

Auricularis

Buccinator

Masseter

Stylohyoid

Orbicularis
oculi

Orbicularis
oris

Mylohyoid

Posterior belly
of digastric

Stylopharyngeus

Cricothyroid

Anterior belly
of digastric

Middle
constrictor
of pharynx

20 weeks

Inferior constrictor
of pharynx

Platysma

FIG 5.7 Muscles from the pharyngeal arches migrate up to form the tongue, the jaw opening/
closing muscles, and the muscles of facial expression. Muscles that move the eyeball arise
in situ and represent a cephalic fusion of movement imperatives. *Adapted from Larsen 1993.*

strength and neurological coordination needed to lift the head with the body.
Only at 6 months is the baby able to elevate the head from the floor when
lying supine. At 8 months a baby is able to sit steadily with no support, yet
it takes another 2 or 3 months for the baby to turn its head without falling
over (Illingworth 1990).

Head on neck control is essential to all movement patterns. It is the supra-hyoid region acting with the suboccipital region that facilitates this crossing from flexion to extension of the head on neck. To extend the head on the neck, muscles such as the SCM, in conjunction with the suboccipital muscles, act with muscles that stabilize the hyoid. The neuromuscular patterning of this righting reaction must be complex as it takes the baby so long to master it.

In summary, a bilateral para-axial ring of contractility has been proposed. Contractility courses around the body, with the left and right domains crossing in the pelvic floor and the jaw/tongue/suboccipital region. This whole person perspective on bending forward and backward runs counter to most current research that attempts to name a muscle or joint as the source of dysfunction. Not only are the dorsal and ventral domains intrinsically melded together, but also this contractility is not isolated from the L-CF that acts as its shape antagonist. The only way to really understand the neuromuscular system is via the concept of 'tune', which is discussed when the archetypal postures are described in Chapter 11.

REFERENCES

Aiello L, Dean C 1990 An introduction to human evolutionary anatomy. Academic Press, London

Beach, P 2007 The contractile field – a new model of human movement, Part 1. Journal of Bodywork and Movement Therapies 11(4):308–317

Blechschmidt E, Gasser R 1978 Biokinetics and biodynamics of human differentiation. Thomas, Illinois

Bogduk N 1997 Clinical anatomy of the lumbar spine and sacrum, 3rd edn. Churchill Livingstone, Edinburgh

Cochard L 2002 Netter's atlas of human embryology. Saunders, Philadelphia

Illingworth R 1990 Basic developmental screening 0–4 years, 5th edn. Blackwell, Oxford

Kent G 1992 Comparative anatomy, 7th edn. Mosby, St Louis

Larsen W 1993 Human embryology. Churchill Livingstone, New York

Liem K, Bemis W, Walker W, Grande L 2001 Functional anatomy of the vertebrates; an evolutionary perspective, 3rd edn. Harcourt, Fort Worth

Maciocia G 1998 A manual of acupuncture. Churchill Livingstone, London, p 496

Schoenwolf G, Bleyl S, Brauer P et al 2008 Larsen's human embryology, 4th edn. Churchill Livingstone, New York

Helical contractile field (H-CF) 6

From the CF perspective, humans have uniquely exploited the potential of helical biodynamics. Our bipedal gait pattern employs it, our ability to project force at a distance employs it, and our brain's complexity employs helical biodynamics to network our hemispheres together in a manner that no other animal has approached.

For centuries, Western medicine has been associated with the caduceus symbol, a Greek magic wand that is a short staff entwined by two snakes. The snakes cross the midline of the staff five to seven times as they wind their way up, with the eyes of the snakes always illustrated. The concept of contractility coursing around the body does remind me of the caduceus symbol so I will describe the helical contractile field (H-CF) from the root of the body up toward the eyes. The H-CF is emergent from the interplay of the dorso/ventro contractile field (D/V-CF) and the lateral contractile field (L-CF). It uses muscles from both those fields but combines them into helical patterns of neuromuscular contraction that are whole-organism in scope. Contractility wraps around the body, repeatedly crossing the ventral and dorsal midline. Like the caduceus symbol the H-CF is a composite of a left and right contractile helix. The conceptual apexes of the H-CF are the eyes and the dens of C2; contractility then wraps around the torso with the nipples and genital tip as embedded nodal regions.

Muscles that are similarly *obliquely* orientated are considered to be participants of this field. Whole-organism functional movements, like gait and throwing, exhibit a seamless diagonal interplay between the left and right domains of the H-CF. All the primary muscles that link the torso to the proximal ends of the long limb bones fit this oblique criterion so I suggest there is a deep affinity between the limbs and the H-CF. This theme will be developed in the chapter on the Limb-CF.

Whole-body twists can be described and I will do this later in the text. However, most of the time, this field is neurologically and biomechanically complex with subsections of the patterning employed in the creative movement of everyday life.

93

DOI: 10.1016/B978-0-7020-3109-0.00011-0

EVOLUTIONARY PERSPECTIVE

Bipedalism presented a complex biomechanical challenge to our tetrapod-derived body as it involved converting a lateral pull of the caudal body into a rotary drive of the pelvic girdle. To demonstrate these issues, imagine I stand upright and side-bend my body repeatedly left and right – eventually I will create a small hole in the ground, but I will not move forwards. A movement pattern used by fish and adopted by tetrapods, and successfully employed for 500 million years, needed a major revision if it was to work for us.

Creating a waist that facilitated contra-rotation of hips and shoulders was necessary for biomechanically efficient bipedal gait. Waists are a particularly human characteristic that all societies appreciate aesthetically. I have come to think that throwing is as fundamental a human activity as walking and running, and that they evolved in biomechanical tandem. Only humans have evolved the ability to over-arm throw accurately. Throwing allows the projection of force from a distance. I cannot imagine an evolutionary scenario that would lead to our overwhelming impact on this planet that did not involve throwing. A throw involves a twist and extension of the upper body on the lower during the wind-up, with a recoil twist and flexion on the throw. A straight shaft such as a spear adds further complexity, as it needs to be pointing toward the prey as this whole-organism twist takes place below. Therefore, the wrist and hand needed to be uncoupled from the twist of the torso otherwise the spear would lose its forward directionality. Subtle changes in the shape of the hamate, a wrist bone at the base of the little finger, allowed a new movement in our hands, ulnar opposition. When you flex your fingers toward the palm they move obliquely toward the base of the thumb, thus allowing a squeezing grip that is essential in throwing and clubbing (Wilson 1999). Concurrently, freeing the wrist and fingers aided signing, a cultural knowledge that some think is a vital precursor to language. Silent signing tactics between participants would have been essential to a successful hunt.

Helical dynamics became whole-organism in scope with upper body twists becoming as imperative to survival as lower body twists. Our lineage has specialized in the exploitation of neurologically challenging helical field biodynamics.

EMBRYOLOGICAL PERSPECTIVE

In principle I trace the origin of this field right back to the mammalian embryonic cleavage pattern, that is, the first divisions of the fertilized egg. Rotational holoblastic cleavage is unique to mammals and, I speculate, has added a rotational dynamic to the core patterning of their development. Rotating the early cleavage planes of mammals is not just an interesting fact, rather it has created a potential for rotary biodynamics that I think our species has literally run with.

You are born with the basic muscular orientation needed for twisting movements, but neurologically, it is not yet coherently patterned across the midline, as the nervous system is not mature enough to process the complex shape changes and weight shifts involved in twisting. However, babies need to master twisting because floor-to-sitting transitions, and sitting-to-standing transitions require it. Walking, running, and throwing mark further sophistication of the H-CF.

FIELD DESCRIPTION

In the real world, the H-CF is a constantly morphing activity that coils and recoils the shape of the body. Oblique fibers pass their pull across the midlines to fibers of the same oblique direction on the contralateral side of the body, usually with a change of fascial depth. The summation of this pattern is a contralateral twisting of the eyes and head, shoulders and pelvis. The essence of this field, sans limbs for conceptual clarity, is depicted below, for the right domain of the H-CF.

I model the left and right domains of the H-CF as summating at a nodal point on the caudal body – these wraps of contractility are so important that their point of singularity must also be biologically important. Conceptually, this field will helix up from the genital tip, here modelled as the caudal singularity of the left and right domains of the H-CFs. The whole urogenital complex is derived from 'intermediate' mesoderm. I have come to associate the word 'intermediate' with helical biodynamics. Any description of our body will involve dorsal/ventral, and a left/right lateral. Intermediate to these primary domains are structures and functions that emerge from the interplay of the primary domains. Where the dorsal body meets the lateral body, where the lateral body meets the ventral body – these intermediate zones that negotiate between primary domains appear to be rich in helical biodynamics. Later in the chapter on acupuncture I will come back to this notion when I consider some of the acupuncture meridians of TCM.

During early embryology (weeks 4–7) the genital region is described as being 'indifferent' in that both sexes have a similar external appearance. A midline genital tubercle emerges that forms the genital tip of both sexes, whilst to the left and right of it, the genital swellings emerge that will form the labia majora or the scrotum. Pioneer muscle cells that have migrated into the pelvic floor at this early stage in development form a pattern that is common to both sexes. Medical students learn the mnemonic 'S2,3,4 keeps the 3Ps off the floor' (penis, poo, and pee) because S2, S3, and S4 innervate the anal sphincter, urethral sphincter, and cause erection. These nerves innervate the muscles of the pelvic floor, such as the bulbospongiosus and the ischiocavernosus that we use in sex. From a sensitive singularity, the genital tip, the H-CF will course up, via the perineal body and the levator ani complex toward the pelvic crests and the inguinal region, to emerge as bigger muscles that can twist the torso.

Like the caduceus wand, contractility emerges to pass either dorsal or ventral to the midline, with the intervertebral discs and vertebral bodies to represent the rod. As can be seen in Figure 6.1, a (left) deep dorsal body-wall muscle that looks quadrilateral in shape, the quadratus lumborum, emerges. It is composed of two obliquely offset fiber directions. When the two oblique fiber directions contract together, this muscle is a powerful (left) side-bending muscle. In this modelling exercise I use only one fiber direction, that of lateral

95

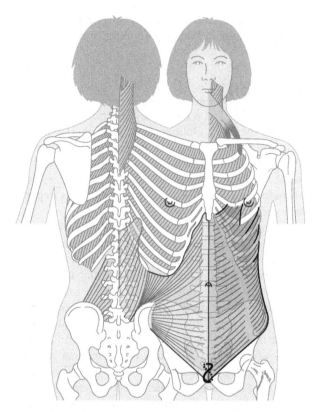

FIG 6.1   The human body divided in the mid-coronal plane like a duck in China town
The wrap of contractility around the body is clearly evident. *Adapted from Beach 2007.*

to medial obliquely upward. From an origin along the iliac crest, muscle fiber courses up and medially to the tips of the transverse process of the lumbar spine and the thoracolumbar fascia. The transverse processes are stout lateral projections of the vertebrae that are the control levers for rotary dynamics. Muscle fibers from the intertransversarii and multifidus muscles will continue fiber direction up to the midline.

The field continues as the (right) serratus posterior inferior, an external muscle of the body-wall. Now we encounter a wrap of body-wall contractile tissue that carries on the oblique superio/lateral fiber direction. The contralateral (right) quadratus lumborum contributes via its other set of oblique muscle fibers. The internal oblique and internal intercostals carry this wrap on and around the (right) body-wall toward the ventral midline. At the ventral midline the wrap of tissue that was internal again decussates to carry on as the (left) external obliques, the (left) external intercostals and the (left) scalene posterior that carries on the fiber pull to the suboccipital region, conceptually coning upward to the dens of C2. The scaleni courses from the first and second ribs to the transverse processes of C2–C6; as mentioned above, the transverse processes are the bony control levers for vertebrate rotation. So muscle dynamics that have coursed around the body-wall end up concentrating a massive rotary force on the cervical vertebrae

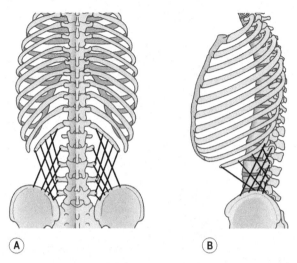

FIG 6.2   The quadratus lumborum A deep muscle with two principal fiber directions.

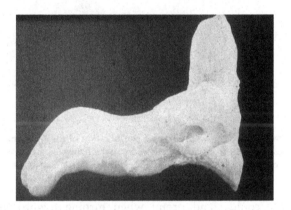

FIG 6.3   Cervical 2 Note the uprightness of the dens. The helical field is modelled as decussating left to right (and vice versa) about the dens.

below the dens of C2. Both the left and right helical field converge on this upright pivot of bone at C2 to blend twisting imperatives, in this way allowing the lower body to rotate in one direction whilst the head can de-couple to rotate in another.

I model the H-CF as decussating around the dens and changing laterality again, emerging as the contralateral (right) sternocleidomastoid (SCM). The spinal root of the accessory nerve supplies the SCM (and the upper fibers of the trapezius). In virtually all cases, the left-brain controls the right muscula-ture, and vice versa – a single decussation across the midline. Interestingly, the nerves that innervate the SCM are described as being double decussated, meaning nerve fibers cross the midline not once but twice. Willoughby and Anderson (1984) noticed in their examination of 100 stroke victims how one side of the body, including the trapezius, could be paralyzed but the SCM on

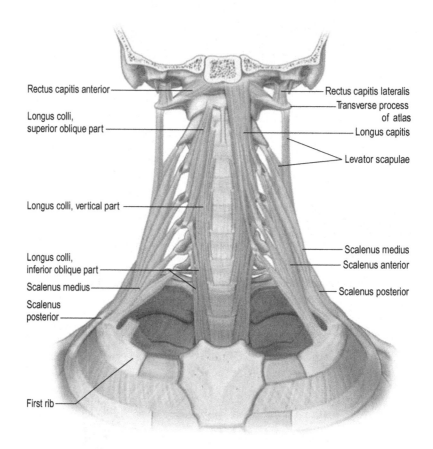

Rectus capitis anterior

Longus colli, superior oblique part

Longus colli, vertical part

Longus colli, inferior oblique part

Scalenus medius

Scalenus posterior

First rib

Rectus capitis lateralis

Transverse process of atlas

Longus capitis

Levator scapulae

Scalenus medius

Scalenus anterior

Scalenus posterior

FIG 6.4 The scalenes are the embryological continuation of the trilaminar body-wall muscles They course obliquely up to insert on the transverse processes of C3–C6. Helical dynamics are blended at the dens of C2. *Adapted from Standring 2008.*

that same side could stand proud when turning toward the damaged hemisphere.

This unusual double decussation allows the SCM to participate in whole-body twists, or to act counter to that twist, as in a spear throw. So the SCM acts as a default righting and visual tracking mechanism. This uniquely complex, slightly spiralized (Williams 1995), neurologically doubly decussed muscle is able to participate in all the CFs. Each field has crossed the midline about three times and has repeatedly changed depth as it courses up in a unified oblique fiber direction.

Cranially, I embed in this field the six muscles that control the eye as they represent the cephalic summit of the neuromuscular system. The lateral rectus has a special affinity with the L-CF, but otherwise they act as a whole to move the eyeball. As whole-body wraps of muscle can so quickly and complexly distort a three-dimensional body shape, the eyes and the otic balance organs are profoundly neurologically coupled to keep you upright.

For example, if I stand and close my eyes I can confidently flex and extend my torso quite quickly. My neurology has enough input from my ears and calf muscles to keep me upright. Likewise, I could rapidly side-bend left/

right with eyes shut, confident that I can stay standing. However, if I close my eyes and try to repeatedly twist up and to the right top quadrant, followed by twisting down and to the left bottom quadrant – now that gets difficult and can quickly lead to a fall. The eyes, with their intermediate placement on the sensory platform, and their ball and socket arrangement are ideally suited and placed to participate in managing complex, twisted shape changes.

THE SPINAL GEARBOX

What I plan to do now is to introduce what I call an 'archetypal twist' that has a 'spinal gearbox' embedded in it. I describe this example of a twist as it is whole-organism in scope following deeply embedded functional anatomy. To do this, I need to explain how the lumbar spine can act as a gearbox that facilitates or inhibits movement patterns. However, the story starts with a quick look at weight distribution patterns.

If you stand and bend forward, where is your weight shifted to in your feet? Is it best to let your weight move toward the toes or backward toward the heel? And what does 'best' mean in this context? I suggest a functional/ safety take on this question. As a baby and child you fall a lot, in old age falling again becomes a real risk. Once you are bipedally stable, falling is bad news. As an adult if you bend forward you are taking 20 or more kilograms with you, so falling is inevitable unless you take weight back onto the heels – the 'easy' way to move as energy is conserved; the same applies when extending the body whilst standing. You have to move weight forward toward the toes or face the real risk of falling backward. These are fundamental 'righting reactions' that we have all learnt, often painfully, as kids. What if, from standing you side-bend to the left? Now which is the easy way to move? Do you want to shift weight to the left foot (ipsilateral), or the right foot (contralateral)? I vote for the right foot as, again, you have moved 20+ kg to the left and you need to transfer weight contralaterally. Contralateral weight transfer makes life 'easy' by maximizing stability and minimizing muscular cost. Let us try another one. Again standing, twist your torso and face to the left as if to hear somebody behind you. You are allowed to move your feet but not completely lift one. Turning to the left do you want to shift weight to your left foot, your right foot, or keep weight central? If you turned your head less than about 30 degrees (pure rotation of the head and C1 on the dens of C2) weight central is the way to go. Bigger twists always involve spinal side-bending – although you are turning to the left your caudal spine is side-bending to the right. Biomechanically, when you side-bend a lordotic spine it rotates contralaterally – a coupled movement. I find it 'easy' when twisting around to the left to stand on the left leg with the right foot up on the toes and a little turned in. Weight shift left counters the side-bending right of the lumbar spine, and rotation left is eased by creating a pivot (left leg) that allows the right pelvis to twist via the lifting up onto the toes of the right foot. In summary: forward bending – take weight back in the feet; backward bending – take weight forwards in the feet; side-bending – take weight to the contralateral foot; when twisting – take weight to the ipsilateral foot.

Now for the gearbox part of this story. It is a story about the developmental relationship between side-bending, flexion/extension, and rotation. You can flex or extend your spine as 'pure' movements as no other vector need be biomechanically coupled. In contrast, if you tip your pelvis into side-bending, vertebrae near the apex of the side-bending vector will also squirm and twist in an attempt to rotate away. This is a spinal coupled movement that has been studied for at least 80 years. For many of those years, debates raged back and forth about which way vertebrae twisted when the spinal column was side-bent. Some studies showed that when the spine was side-bent right the lumbar vertebrae twisted right; other studies contradicted this and found side-bending right was coupled with left rotation, or no rotation at all (Lovett et al, as referenced in Gracovetsky 1988). Gradually a theoretical consensus has arisen.

Much of the confusion came about because it was not realized how important the degree of lumbar flexion or extension was to the torque that is generated by side-bending. When the lumbar spine is extended into a lordotic shape, a side-bend left will then subject vertebrae and pelvis to a contralateral twist, in this case to the right. Flexion of the lumbar spine invokes a quite different response. If flexed and side-bent left the lumbar spine and pelvis will want to rotate left (ipsilateral rotation). In effect, a spinal gearbox with a forward and reverse gearing pattern is created via the biomechanics of the facet joints, the intervertebral discs between the vertebrae, and diagonally opposed muscle.

Crocodiles, for example, do not have this reverse gear coupling in their spine. If they crawl into a long narrow box they must try to turn around as they cannot just reverse out. I have seen a video of a 7- or 8-month-old child who has just learnt to sit unaided, but with a slumped, flexed spine. Something attractive was placed in front of the child, her eyes lit up, and she tried to shuffle forward on her sitting bones toward the object. But the harder she tried to move forward the further away from the object of desire she became. The frustration on the child's face was poignant. A couple of weeks later when a child can sit erect, when she lifts one side of her pelvis up (that is the side-bending), it is coupled to a forward drive of that sitting bone. By sitting up she has found forward gear and can move toward the object of her desire. A lordosis and side-bending is forward gear, lumbar flexion and side-bending is reverse gear. As an adult if you hurt your lower back so that you are unable to stand upright you will find yourself moving painfully forward with small, slow steps. Walking backward would be faster. Likewise, if you are participating in a tug-of-war, you do not pull with a straight back. You round your back, engage reverse and power-up.

I have used these ideas (helical fields, weight shift, and spinal gearbox) to discern an archetypal twist of the body. It goes like this. From standing, reach with both arms and torso up into your right upper quadrant above your head. Importantly, the movement will start with a tilting of the torso to the left, with rotation of the torso right because the lumbar spine is lordotic. Because you are side-bent left and rotated right the easy way to transfer weight is to the right leg. From this top right quadrant follow through and down, crossing the midline. As you move down toward your bottom left quadrant you will keep the left side-bending but your lumbar spine that was extended now becomes flexed. Now the path of ease is left side-bending and left rotation with weight transfer to the left foot.

In the real world, this field is staggeringly complex. The left and right domains of the H-CF are warped and weft together. If both oblique fiber directions contract on one side they are employed as the lateral field. Interweaving these fields is the deep radial field that squeezes and shape manages the body-wall. Out of this complex emerges a number of zones and lines of decussation. Coherent shape control of the body-wall is mediated via these emergent long-axis lines. Decussation primarily occurs at the:

- Dorsal midline
- High point of the erector spinae
- Rib angles
- Linea semilunaris
- High point of the rectus abdominis crest
- Medial margin of the rectus sheath
- Ventral midline.

Embedded within mammalian biodynamics the emergent H-CF is modelled as coalescing at: the eyes, the supra/infra and mental foramina, the canines, the dens of C2, the nipples, the upper and lower limbs, the gonads, and genital tip caudally.

REFERENCES

Beach P 2007 The contractile field: a new model of human movement, part 1. Journal of Bodywork and Movement Therapies 11(4):308–317

Gracovetsky S 1988 The spinal engine. Springer-Verlag Wein, New York

Standring S 2008 Gray's anatomy, 40th edn. Churchill Livingstone, Philadelphia

Williams P 1995 Gray's anatomy, 38th edn. Churchill Livingstone, Edinburgh

Willoughby E, Anderson N 1984 Lower cranial nerve motor function in unilateral vascular lesions of the cerebral hemisphere. British Medical Journal 289:791–794

Wilson F 1999 The hand; how its use shapes the brain, language, and human culture. Vintage Books, New York

Limb contractile fields (Limb-CFs)

7

Limbs both control and empower vertebrate movement. The CF model suggests they are most simply seen as having dorsal and ventral moieties that straddle that part of the body-wall that influences helical biodynamics.

Upper and lower limbs have had 500 million years of divergent functional evolution, therefore important differences exist. Mammalian limbs emerge as limb buds from a transient structure that encircles the embryo called the ectodermal ring (also known as the Wolffian ridge). By following these two lines of enquiry the CF model suggests:

* Limbs emerge from and empower the biodynamics of the H-CF
* Limbs are succinctly modelled as having dorsal and ventral moieties (halves)
* Limb function is built around a series of archetypal postures
* Limbs express themselves via the hands and feet.

In this chapter, the evolution of our limbs will be briefly reviewed, then we will look again at the embryology of the limbs. Once these contexts have been set the muscle fields will be introduced. In Chapter 11 the importance of archetypal postures to limb function is proposed. Looking at limb function from these perspectives has important clinical implications.

For conceptual clarity it is best to model limb function as distinct from the musculature of the torso. Many vertebrate species have lost their limbs so if we are to model movement patterns across vertebrates, rather than referring only to the human form, we need to place limbs in a developmental context. Limbs command their own genetic modules of embryonic development, modules that are common to all vertebrates, and even across phyla. Fly wings employ a genetic cascade that is very similar to the cascade that mammals use (Carroll 2005).

EVOLUTIONARY PERSPECTIVE

Vertebrate shapes that evolved within water became streamlined. Any streamlined body has a tendency to tip and deviate from its line of travel. It may swing from side to side (yaw), rock about its long axis (roll), or deviate

103

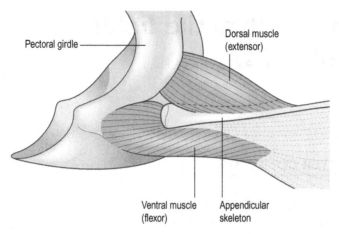

Pectoral girdle

Dorsal muscle (extensor)

Ventral muscle (flexor)

Appendicular skeleton

FIG 7.1 **Note how the dorsal and ventral muscles do not function in one plane** They embrace the borders of the fin; this allows more complex fin movement. *Adapted from Liem et al Functional anatomy of the vertebrates, 3rd edn.© 2001 Brookes/Cole, a part of Cengage Learning, Inc. Reproduced by permission.*

up or down (pitch). These directional deviations are corrected for by fins that are exquisitely positioned (Kardong 1998). Along the ventro-lateral edge of many fish is a 'fin-fold' from which the fins will emerge. Fin musculature is derived from embryonic myomeres (the precursor of muscle) near the base of each fin fold. The migrating myomeres divide into dorsal and ventral moieties (tissue blocks). Dorsal moieties form extensors (abductors, levators, supinators – all these terms are used); ventral moieties form the flexors (adductors, depressors, pronators).

Nearly all fish have pectoral and pelvic girdles that are small and weak as the fins are not propulsive. From an evolutionary perspective, the upper girdle is older, larger, and more complicated than the pelvic girdle. The upper girdle of fish is a composite of bones that are derived from protective scale armour (called dermal bones that have sunk into the body-wall) and endoskeleton bones that have replaced a cartilaginous precursor. The upper girdle is attached to the base of the fish skull and lies immediately behind the gills.

Fins are carefully placed on the body-wall to control movement, and so too are limbs. Terrestrial life demanded a massive increase in the strength and weight of the new limbs, both to lift the body off the substrate and take on propulsive duties.

Over time, amphibians detached the pectoral girdle away from the skull thereby creating a neck of flexible vertebral segments. A stout U-shaped girdle evolved that lost much of the dermal bone (the clavicle is the only girdle dermal bone retained by mammals), replaced by a deeper bracing of endoskeletal elements.

Bipedalism freed the upper girdle from weight-bearing duties; this in turn facilitated feeding with both arms, signing as a proto-language, tool manufacture and use, and throwing via a further exploitation of a waist pre-adapted for bipedal gait. The hand has responded to these evolutionary pressures by staying at a less specialized developmental stage, a process known as paedomorphosis. A baby chimp and baby human have similarly shaped faces and hands that will diverge in proportions later in development, so many human characteristics are paedomorphic. Within this general trend the wrist and hand subtly morphed toward the ability to use more grips for throwing and clubbing.

EMBRYOLOGICAL PERSPECTIVE

Limbs are a late starter in embryology. They first emerge as tiny buds on the ventro-lateral body-wall that, over a developmental period spanning many years, come to represent a large percentage of your total body weight. The CF model places particular emphasis on the fact that limbs are extrusions from the intermediate body-wall of the embryo so, due to this placement, it is suggested that they are deeply embedded within the genesis of whole-organism helical fields.

The key aspects revised here are that limbs are emergent from the Wolffian ridge so are developmentally integrated with the formation of the nose, eyes, ears, nipples, and genital tip. In a sense the hands and feet have become the executive organs for the sensory platform and the genital region. The dense core of the limb bud that will chondrify and later ossify is derived from a migration of cells into the limb bud from the intermediate (precursive kidney and coelom) region of the embryonic body. These cells bring with them information that is 'remembered' from earlier positional and inductive histories (Carlson 1994). An example of this memory from another tissue is the development of neurons. New neuronal cells emerge from a nursery deep in the brain and issue forth with birthdays that can be radioactively tagged. These neuronal cells begin a remarkable migration toward the cortex, which can be likened to driving across a continent without a map (Edelman 1992). On the way, cells stop and form relationships with local cells; these neuronal connections are kept as the neuron detaches most of itself to rise again through a brain that is experiencing warp-speed enlargement. So each neuron has a unique experience of the brain as it comes to finally settle in the six-layered cortex. In a similar way I suggest the subtle shape and biomechanical function of bony tissue 'remembers' this early positional relationship with the coelom and the precursive kidneys in particular. This association is not new, as the Chinese medical community has linked the Qi of the Kidneys to the limbs for the past 2000 years.

In contrast, primordial muscle tissue migrates into the limb bud from the dorsal side of the embryo. Muscle precursor cells migrate into the limb bud from the somites and establish a dorsal and ventral moiety. These muscle masses then repeatedly split into the definitive muscles of the limb. Nerve supply reflects this early division into dorsal and ventral muscle masses. Some muscles migrate from their early position so an embryonic extensor muscle may actually have a flexor action in the adult (such as the brachioradialis of the forearm).

Box 7.1 contains a listing of dorso-ventro origin for some major limb muscles (Crafts 1985).

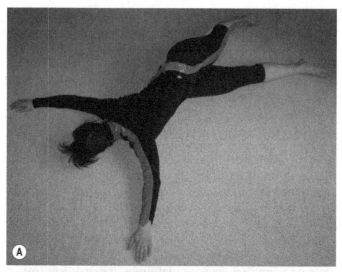

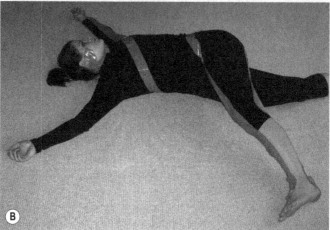

FIG 7.2 The upper and lower limb dorsal and ventral muscle moieties complexly wrap around the torso There are many ways of wrapping this contractility to both the ipsilateral and contralateral arm and leg. Each attempt to visualize one wrap hides another. The wraps of contractility depicted here must interact with the extra-ocular muscles, the sternocleidomastoid (SCM), the dens of C2, then course down the arm, around the torso to the iliac crest, via the psoas and iliacus to the quadriceps group, to the extensors of the foot, then via the ventral moiety muscles on the dorsal surface of the leg back to the pelvic floor. Note that the tape used to depict the wraps of contractility should be about five or six spinal segments wide as this many embryonic segments contribute to each limb bud.

DISCUSSION

Mammalian limbs, in this model, are seen as power amplifiers of helical bio-dynamics. The upper limbs amplify the body's ability to twist the torso from the suboccipital complex to the waist, whereas the lower limb empowers the caudal body to twist from the pelvic floor up. If you throw a stone-age

---

BOX 7.1 Ventral and dorsal muscle mass derivation

Ventral

Upper limb
- Anterior compartment of the arm and forearm, pectoralis major and minor
- The muscles of the palm

Lower limb
- Medial compartment muscles of the thigh
- Posterior compartment muscles of the thigh (except short head of biceps femoris)
- Posterior compartment muscles of the leg
- All muscles on the plantar surface of the foot
- Obturator internus, gemellus superior/inferior, quadratus femoris

Dorsal

Upper limb
- Posterior compartment muscles of the arm and forearm
- Lateral compartment muscles of the forearm and hand
- Deltoid, latissimus dorsi, rhomboids, levator scapulae, serratus anterior, teres major and minor, subscapularis, supraspinatus, infraspinatus

Lower limb
- Anterior compartment muscles of the thigh and leg
- Tensor fascia lata, short head of biceps femoris
- Lateral compartment muscles of the leg
- Muscles of the dorsum of the foot
- Gluteus maximus/medius/minimus, piriformis, iliacus, psoas

---

handaxe with your right hand, your torso will side-bend to the left but twist to the right. The right nipple will be drawn backward with the right arm whereas the left nipple will project forwards. The CF model suggests the nipples mark nodal regions in the body's ability to twist. Recall that the nipple line is that part of the Wolffian ridge that linked the upper limb bud to the lower limb bud. Nipple/breast asymmetries may reflect more than just a local asymmetry as they are emergent from archetypal helical patterns that affect many organs in development and function. For example, there appears to be a link between breast asymmetry and cancer rates (Scutt et al 2006).

The lower limb has traded dexterity for bipedal locomotor duties. The lower limb bud internally rotates and the long axis twists during early development, to become fully cross-legged flexed and ankle dorsiflexed at full term. Post birth the legs assume a partially flexed/abducted posture. With the developmental acquisition of bipedal gait the legs are at first bowed, then a knock-kneed period is normal, ideally then assuming a feet together and knees together with the patella facing forwards posture when standing upright.

BOX 7.2   Muscle courses obliquely from the torso to the limbs

Flexors (right arm)
Quadratus lumborum lateral to medial oblique fibers (right), serratus posterior inferior (left), internal oblique (left), internal intercostals (left), thoracic external intercostals (right), pectoralis major (right), anterior compartment muscles of the arm, forearm and palmar surface of the hand (right)

Extensors (right arm)
Internal oblique (right), external oblique (left), external intercostals (left), trapezius (right), latissimus dorsi (right), rhomboids (right), infraspinatus (right), teres major and minor (right), posterior compartment of the arm and forearm (right)

The internal rotation and long axis twist of the lower limb is important. As described in the embryological chapter, the lower limb acts like a pogo stick due to the coiling of the musculature. Each foot strike stores energy in the ligamentous system that is released with take-off. Walking on your hands is tremendously tiring as the arms do not have this coil/recoil mechanism and their girdles have to be constantly supported by a muscular sling. Even 20 meters hand standing is a huge effort.

REFERENCES

Carlson B 1994 Human embryology and developmental biology. Mosby, St Louis

Carroll SB 2005 Endless forms most beautiful. Weidenfeld & Nicolson, London

Crafts R 1985 A textbook of human anatomy. Churchill Livingstone, New York

Edelman G 1992 Bright air, brilliant fire. Penguin, London

Kardong K 1998 Vertebrates: comparative anatomy, function, evolution, 2nd edn. WCB/McGraw-Hill, Boston

Liem K, Bemis W, Walker W, Grande L 2001 Functional anatomy of the vertebrates: an evolutionary perspective, 3rd edn. Harcourt College Publishers, Fort Worth

Scutt D, Lancaster GA, Manning JT 2006 Breast asymmetry and predisposition to breast cancer. Breast Cancer Research 8:R14

Radial contractile field (R-CF)   8

To preserve spinal length, vertebrates squeeze the torso. Tetrapods employ similar muscles to suck air for respiration. Squeezing and sucking are flip sides of the same coin.

All the contractile fields discussed so far have a common effect on the spine – they will all shorten and eventually buckle the spinal complex. If flexion or extension, lateral flexion left or right, or twisting to the left or to the right are carried too far the spine will kink, a painful condition that can take months to recover from. The radial contractile field (R-CF) has an anti-buckling function by squeezing the body-wall. The gym world calls this 'core strength' or 'core stability.' As well as considering the muscles that squeeze the body-wall, mammals, in particular, have developed the essential ability to suck. Our diaphragm, a muscle that is modelled as participating in the R-CF, acts as a suction pump. We swell as we inhale. The term 'radial' was chosen to describe this increase and decrease in the circumference of the body-wall that squeezing and sucking will create.

The squeezing action of the R-CF is felt during a forced expiration through pursed lips. The spine acts as a braced dorsal structure that this muscular field acts about in its action of squeezing the dorso/ventro and lateral body-wall together. If you imagine squeezing a tube of gel it will exert a pressure on the top and bottom of the tube. What is lost in dorsal/ventral and lateral diameters is added to the longitudinal length of the tube, or increased longitudinal stiffness.

A radial field that acts about the notochordal remnants will cause an elongation and stiffening of the spine. When a field of torso-encircling muscle contracts, intra-cranial, intra-thoracic, and intra-abdominal compartmental pressures rise. The interaction of compartmental pressures determines much of your fundamental body shape. Raised compartmental pressures will seek their release by testing the integrity of the oral/anal sphincters and diaphragmatic/abdominal wall vulnerabilities. Hernias mark the areas in this field where defects are commonly found. Umbilical, inguinal, femoral, diaphragmatic, and intervertebral disc hernias all reduce the body's ability to raise functionally important compartmental pressures.

109

© 2010 Elsevier Ltd / Inc / Bv
DOI: 10.1016/B978-0-7020-3109-0.00013-4

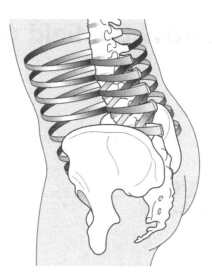

FIG 8.1 Schematic diagram of the radial-CF in the abdomen

The converse of squeezing is sucking. Mammals are hot-blooded animals that are very active so they have evolved a respiratory system that is capable of providing the large-volume gas exchange needed to oxygenate a vigorous body. Mammals, by definition, suckle, so mobile lips that can seal on the nipple and areola, allied with a musculature that can actively suck, are conceptually included in this CF. At the caudal end of the gut tube the external anal ring is also conceptually embedded in this field. The R-CF is intimately linked to visceral function and contributes to the shape of the torso about which the outer layers of the trilaminar body wall and limbs act.

EMBRYOLOGICAL PERSPECTIVE

The radial field represents the deep layer of the trilaminar body-wall. As mesoderm is drawn laterally/ventrally with embryonic folding it enters morphogenic fields that split it into three muscle layers that each experience a different fiber direction imperative. The transversus abdominis undergoes the most extreme fiber orientation change from longitudinal, as is the erector spinae, to roughly transverse, dorsal to ventral.

The transversus abdominis interdigitates with the insertion of the diaphragm on the costal cartilage margin. The diaphragm originates in the neck region of the embryo as the septum transversum, which is a mesodermal bridge into which the early liver grows. As it develops, four embryonic structures contribute to it. Differential growth of the embryo as the brain ascends and the heart descends pulls the septum transversum down into the thorax, dragging the left and right phrenic nerves (C3, C4, C5) with it. As the septum transversum descends it appropriates inner thoracic wall mesoderm to contribute to its muscularity. The crura of the diaphragm are probably derived from mesoderm associated with the foregut at the level of L1, L2, and L3. Another source of the diaphragm is the pleuroperitoneal

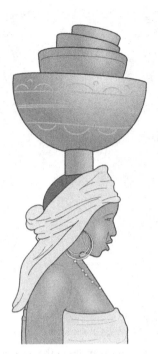

FIG 8.2 The R-CF is employed in breathing and lifting and, as in this remarkable example of balance, acts as an anti-buckling mechanism. Carrying a weight in this manner is extraordinarily biomechanically efficient. In contrast, the Western backpack with no head harness is a biomechanically ungracious, inefficient way to carry weight.

membranes that are associated with the separation of the pleural cavities from the peritoneal cavity.

All the three layers of the mesodermal body wall are said to be induced by the ectoderm, and I suspect, the deep layer of being also induced by a patent endoderm – the underlying viscera. There is a syndrome called 'prune belly' that afflicts about 1 in 40 000 babies. The vast majority are males who are born with abdominal wall muscle defects associated with a variety of urogenital, gastrointestinal, and musculoskeletal malformations. The syndrome appears to afflict the male urogenital system and this abnormality then affects the development of the low abdominal wall, in turn causing multiple organ abnormalities. Organs and muscles co-develop so that at critical moments abnormality in one domain can trigger a cascade of developmental abnormalities across multiple tissue domains (Carlson 1994).

EVOLUTIONARY PERSPECTIVE

The diaphragm is a muscle that is found in precursive form as the septum transversum of fish and with terrestriality as the pulmonary muscle we are familiar with. Mammals have moved the diaphragm to be post-lung and pre-hepatic. This field is intimately linked to visceral function and contributes to the shape of the torso about which the outer layers of the trilaminar body-wall and limbs act.

111

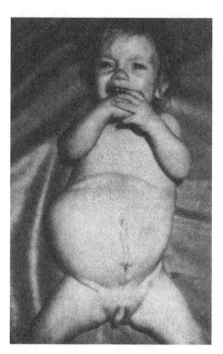

FIG 8.3 Prune belly syndrome affects males in the majority of cases It is associated with urogenital, gastrointestinal, and musculoskeletal abnormalities. The abdominal muscles are affected and the ribs often outflare. *From Wigglesworth and Singer 1991, with permission.*

FIELD DESCRIPTION

The R-CF is modelled as being embryologically derived from voluntary muscles around the mouth and face, then encircling the torso, to the voluntary muscles that encircle the anus caudally. Mesoderm and endoderm meet at these orifices. Participating structures include:

- The sense organs modelled to be embedded in this field are the lips and the external anus.
- Buccinator, Latin for the trumpeter as it expels air in blowing and acts during mastication of food.
- Orbicularis oris and orbicularis oculi are both muscles that can be seen to contract on strong squeezing exertions.
- The platysma is a superficial muscle that blends with the orbicularis oris that rings the mouth. It fires with sudden inhalations and in straining lifts. Here is an example of a muscle that is superficial but is functionally linked with the deeper muscles of core stabilization. Interestingly, it is derived from a muscle called the constrictor colli that is particularly well developed in fish as it forms the main muscles of the water-breathing pump. The muscle partially encircles the neck from the hyoid region to the ventral midline in amphibians. It is thought most of the muscles of mammalian facial expression are derived from the constrictor colli as it is innervated by the facial nerve, inserts on the skin, and is known to migrate to the face where it splits repeatedly (Kardong 1998).

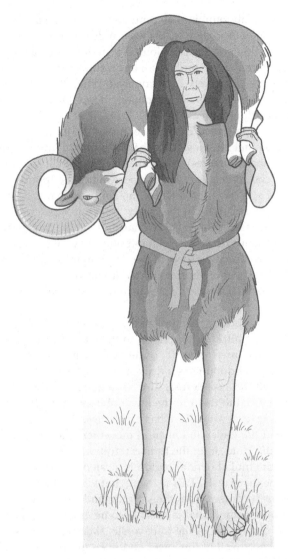

FIG 8.4 Transporting resources was a functional need for all people until recently
It activates the R-CF. *Adapted from Beach 2007.*

- Muscles that are involved in a Valsalva maneuver that brace the torso and throat before a heavy lift are modelled as R-CF. The Valsalva maneuver (named after Antonio Maria Valsalva, a 17th-century physician and anatomist with a special interest in the ear) is a forced exhalation against a closed glottis. Intra-thoracic and intra-abdominal pressures rise thus causing a transient rise in blood pressure, followed by a bradycardia. A Valsalva maneuver is unavoidable with defecation and weightlifting.
- The anterior scalene (embryologically the deepest of the three scalenes) continues the R-CF. Separating the scalenes out like this aids conceptual clarity but these three muscles must function together.

113

- The transversus abdominis is continuous with the costal origin of the diaphragm. The diaphragm is, likewise, a deep muscle and both share the same insertion and are functionless without the other. For example, if the pelvic organs have prolapsed, one's ability to lift weights or breathe strongly is severely compromised. When the R-CF is compromised the spine is not adequately hoop braced in movement and is liable to buckling injury.
- Respiration is a patterned interplay between the thoracic wall muscles and the abdominal muscles. Both share a common innervation (ventral rami of the thoracic nerves) and both are embryologically derived from the same fascial layers. Within the inner wall of the thorax the deepest layer of muscle is the intercostal intimi, a muscle that is described as being patchy, particularly in the upper thorax. It is patchy because some of the muscle was appropriated to contribute to the muscular ring that pulls the tendinous dome of the diaphragm down within the thorax. Note that the contractile aspect of the diaphragm is near vertical as compared with the more horizontal tendinous dome.
- Other endothoracic muscles in this field are the sternocostalis and the subcostals.
- The transversus abdominis muscle spans the abdomen from the lateral margins of the quadratus lumborum to the iliac crest, the inguinal ligament and the inferior border of the costal cartilages of ribs T6–T12. The transversus abdominis is a deep muscle in its costal area, gradually diving through the aponeurosis of the internal and external oblique, to become superficial to them in the lower abdominal wall. The Chinese exercise and martial art culture has for thousands of years stressed the importance of the lower abdomen in movement patterns. The Dantian (also called the Hara or, in the Indian tradition a similar concept has been called the mula bhanda) region is located below the navel, about level with the iliac crests. This is the region where the transversus abdominis, as it courses from the sternum and ribs toward the pubis, emerges from a deep fascial layer to become, briefly, a superficial muscle. The emergence of the transversus abdominis to a superficial layer of the body-wall in the lower abdomen means it can pull the trilaminar body wall inward toward the center, exerting a maximum push upward on the viscera, hence the dome of the diaphragm, with a minimum downward pressure on the pelvic floor.
- The entire pelvic floor is dynamically interlinked with the diaphragm and the transversus abdominis as a pressurized intra-abdominal compartment. The perineal body and the external muscles of the anus are embedded in the R-CF. Our bipedal gait has required a strengthening of this area.

DISCUSSION

Activities such as singing, shouting, foot stomping, hopping, jumping, lifting and pushing, rising from the floor, etc. are all rich in the biodynamics that will employ the R-CF. These activities are amongst the core suite of functional evolutionary activities. And these are activities that our desk-bound society neglects. Many of our current exercise programs are analogous to junk food (calories with no complex nutrients) in that they bulk up individual muscles but do little toward a whole organism functional integration of the musculature. For example, gym bicycle riding will not require or contribute to a robust and neurologically complex R-CF. Nor will sitting whilst exercising, a quite bizarre posture to exercise from. Likewise, the use of a blood pressure cuff to measure abdominal hollowing and 'core' muscle activation is unlikely to help develop or support functional movement patterns. From the perspective of the CF the core muscles cannot be structurally or functionally divorced from the body whole. As I suggest in the chapter on archetypal postures (Ch. 11), it is an appreciation of the crucial role these postures play to our biomechanical tune that is important.

Resource transport has been a function of our lifestyles for hundreds of generations. The *Homo* lineage developed a wide gathering and hunting range, the products of which would have been transported back to the camp. It is no accident that worldwide, simple baskets with a forehead strap have been employed to carry. Loading the forehead will transfer the acquired weight to the entire spine that will then stiffen in response. Nepalese porters regularly carry their body weight in produce using this simple harnessing technique. The Western backpack does not load the R-CF appropriately. In a manner similar to the righting reactions, if 20 kg is placed on the shoulders and back the body will attempt to move 20 kg forward, thus placing a shear strain on the junction between the neck and thorax. Backpack manufacturers would be advised to incorporate a lightweight harness from the base of the pack that then has a webbing for the head. It could be removable and used only when the pack is heavy. With modern materials the harness would be both light and effective. Biomechanical efficiency would increase so one could walk further with less metabolic cost and the likelihood of chronic neck/shoulder pain would be reduced.

Load carrying on the head is another way of carrying loads very efficiently when the terrain will allow it. Up to 40% of one's body weight can be placed on the head basket with almost no metabolic cost to the carrier. This remarkable efficiency is probably due to a smoother gait pattern that the added weight seems to encourage.

The R-CF compresses the viscera. If the intestines are inflamed they are able to override the squeezing body-wall muscles. One is unable to develop a strong bracing of the torso because of the pain signals fed into the neurological system from the visceral inflammation. Visceral shape and function profoundly affect the ability of the R-CF to both squeeze and suck.

REFERENCES

Beach P 2007 The contractile field: a new model of human movement, part 1. Journal of Bodywork and Movement Therapies 11(4):308–317

Carlson B 1994 Human embryology and developmental biology. Mosby, St Louis

Kardong K 1998 Vertebrates: comparative anatomy, function, evolution, 2nd edn. WCB/McGraw-Hill, Boston

Wigglesworth J, Singer D 1991 Textbook of fetal and perinatal pathology. Blackwell Scientific, Oxford

Chiralic contractile field (C-CF) 9

To model human movement solely from the perspective of the muscles of the body-wall and limbs is patently inadequate from both a theoretical and a clinical perspective. The asymmetric musculature of the cardiovascular system and the gastrointestinal system are core contributors to our movement patterns.

The CFs described thus far use body-wall and limb musculature to coherently change the shape of the body via the interaction of primary movement patterns. However, a conceptual space needs to be created within which another category of contractility can be tentatively modelled. This field, which I call the chiralic CF (C-CF), is structurally and functionally quite different to the CFs described in the preceding chapters. The C-CF is abstracted from the visceral muscle that powers the peristaltic movement of the gastrointestinal tract (GIT) and the pulsatile movement of the cardiovascular system (CVS).

SYMMETRY V. ASYMMETRY

There are many structural and functional differences between the voluntary somatic muscle tissue of the body-wall and limbs compared with the involuntary visceral muscle tissue. On reflection, there is one difference between the two categories of contractility that is of primordial importance that I chose to emphasize in naming this CF: the profound relationship between the bilaterally symmetrical body-wall musculature versus the handed nature of the visceral musculature that empowers the GIT and the CVS.

The word 'chiral' is derived from the Greek word *kheir*, meaning hand. In the biochemical context it refers to a three-dimensional form that is non-superimposable on its mirror image, that is, it has a topological handedness. Not surprisingly, our hands are an example of chirality in that they are mirror images of each other, but using a mirror you cannot rotate your left hand to superimpose it on your right hand. Sliding one hand on top of the

117

other will not superimpose them, nor will turning one hand over and super-imposing them as now the front and back are reversed – hence the hands are handed. Or to put it another way, a right hand will never fit properly into a left-hand glove.

Chirality thus concerns the handedness of structures, a subject that has turned out to be biologically very important. For reasons that the initiated can only speculate about, the molecules of life have a profound affinity for one 'hand' over the other. In 2001 the Nobel Prize in Chemistry was awarded to William Knowles, Ryoji Noyori, and K. Barry Sharpless for their pioneering work in developing the ability to catalyze important reactions so that only one of the two mirror images of a chiral molecule is produced (called an enantiomer). The importance of chirality had became apparent when the thalidomide disaster of the 1960s was traced to the right-handed form of the molecule (also known as the D-form) being an effective hypnotic for morning sickness, but the left-handed form (the L-form) in this case proved to be a teratogen by causing the birth defects that ruined so many young lives. As is usual in biology, the cause of this tragedy proved to be more complex because it was then found that the 'safe' D-thalidomide is not stable and can convert to the teratogenic L-thalidomide in water (McManus 2002). Chirality had proved itself to be a matter of life and death, hence the need to be able to produce either the left- or right-handed form of a chiral molecule that was biochemically stable.

Living organisms, drug receptors, chiral molecules, and many enzymes are able to recognize chirality. To comprehend why this may be so, imagine meeting a colleague and shaking their hand. If both of you present your right hands in the conventional way the mutual grip is strong and familiar. However, quite bizarrely, if your colleague has just returned from another chiral universe and presents their left hand to your right hand the handshake grip will be most unfamiliar and unreciprocated. Biological chemistry also favours one grip over the other, as chiral molecules feel for their mutually compatible docking stations.

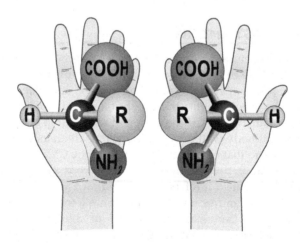

FIG 9.1   Molecules and hands are chiral structures *Courtesy of NASA Astrobiology Institute.*

The relationship between symmetry and asymmetry is a major preoccupation of scientific cosmology, mathematics, and biology – it is a relationship that each of us has embodied. We associate good form and health with an external bilateral symmetry but internally asymmetry is the norm as the embryonic cardiac tube twists to form a loop to the right, and our intestines coil counterclockwise 270 degrees in development (Larsen 1993). The visceral organs are not symmetrical but they are handed. The handedness of the visceral organs can be swapped so that, for example, the apex of the heart may point to the right instead of the left, a condition that is called dextrocardia. When the other visceral organs such as the liver, stomach, and spleen also swap sides (situs inversus) there are often no apparent symptoms. If dextrocardia occurs without a general situs inversus then the chances of organ abnormality are dramatically increased.

Much of the groundwork for the C-CF has been introduced via the chapters on the evolution of body-plans and the embryological development of the coelom. A true coelom (i.e. one that develops within the mesodermal layer) became essential to the evolution of movement in many body-plans including ours. A coelom created the tube within a tube arrangement that semi-isolated our gut and blood vessel movement from our body-wall movement. The outer leaf of mesoderm is called the somatic, from which all the muscles we rub and stretch in manual therapy are derived, all of which are ideally bilaterally symmetrical. For every named muscle on the left we have a right counterpart.

The inner leaf is called the splanchnic; from this mesodermal layer the visceral musculature will coalesce. Mammals divide the intervening coelom into three primary, cavities: the pericardial, the pleural, and the peritoneal. The importance of the muscle derived from the splanchnopleure to our movement patterns cannot be underestimated. When the relationship between these two layers of muscle goes awry it can have devastating consequences.

When the remnants of the coelom are compromised in their ability to allow slip between the body-wall musculature and the viscera, the effects on one's ease of movement are dramatic. An Olympic athlete suffering from pericarditis, pleurisy, or peritonitis will need modern medical treatment pronto as the highly trained muscles of the torso and limbs are predicated on a degree of disassociation from the visceral core. The coelom is as important to movement now as it was 500 MYA when an innovation in body-plans created the tube within a tube construction that most animal life on Earth today employs.

The C-CF is modelled around two core visceral movements – pulsatile and peristaltic. To single out the pulsatile and peristaltic from the whole gamut of visceral movement is obviously a simplification but it does begin the theoretical contemplation of the relationship of the somatic to the splanchnic. My aim here is to create a conceptual space where we may consider how the asymmetric visceral musculature contributes to movement as the usual remit of those that study and attend dysfunctions of movement often extends only to the external muscles, bones, and joints; however, the movement of our gut tube and the blood pressures created by our heart underlie all the movements of our external life.

THE PERICARDIUM

The pulsating heart is encased by a structure called the pericardium. It is a thin sac that surrounds the heart. The pericardium has two layers, one of which is intimately connected to the heart, whilst the outer layer is attached to the sternum, the proximal ends of the major heart vessels, the top of the diaphragm, and the mediastinum. Between the layers is a microscopic film of serous fluid that acts to reduce friction between the pulsating heart and the chest cavity. The pericardium is a tough structure that anchors the heart to stop it writhing like a high-pressure garden hose in your chest, and it will resist the swelling of the heart during high blood pressure events.

Pericarditis is an inflammation between the layers that may arise slowly or suddenly, usually felt as chest pain described as sharp and stabbing. The pain may radiate to the back, scapula, neck, or arm. Pericarditis is often positional, where lying on one's back increases the pain and shortness of breath whereas bending forward usually relieves it.

THE PLEURAE

A closed invaginated sac surrounds each lung. The visceral pleura (the surface attached to the lung) slide on the parietal pleura (the surface attached to the chest wall, diaphragm, and the mediastinal contents) via a serous pleural fluid. The pleurae allow the lungs to move within the chest with little friction, and surface tension within the pleural cavity holds the lung closely to the internal chest wall. Hence large excursions of the rib cage will change the shape of the lungs.

When the pleural cavity is ruptured or inflamed (called pleurisy or pleuritis) the symptoms usually include severe chest pain that is often worse when breathing in, an inability to take a deep breath, a shortness of breath, and if the cause is infective, fever/chills will accompany this distress.

THE PERITONEUM

The peritoneum is similar in form and function to the other remnants of the coelom. It is a bilaminar serous membrane that contains a slippery fluid that encloses most of the abdominal contents. Visceral organs are tethered to the wall of the torso by mesenteries that are derived from the peritoneum. Blood vessels and nerves enter the viscera via these mesenteries. Each organ has a range of normal physiological movement that can be contemplated only with reference to the other viscera that closely constrain it.

Peritonitis, i.e. inflammation of the peritoneum, may affect the whole peritoneum or it may be isolated to an area as a pus-filled abscess. Rupture or obstruction anywhere along the GIT is the most common pathway for the entry of an infectious agent. Peritonitis causes acute severe pain in all or part of the abdomen; the abdominal wall muscles contract to a board-like rigidity, the abdomen becomes swollen and bloated, there is nausea, vomiting and sweating, the skin is pale and clammy, and peristalsis stops. It is a serious condition that requires antibiotics and often surgical intervention.

THE PULSATILE DOMAIN OF THE C-CF

During early embryogenesis the embryonic disc laminates with a distinct ectoderm, a mesoderm, and an endoderm. At the rostral end of this flattened pear-shaped disc is a pinching together of the germ layers that is called the buccopharyngeal membrane, which marks the site of the future mouth. Cells that will contribute to the formation of the heart gather in a cardiogenic region that is rostral and lateral to the future mouth. With embryonic folding the heart primordium is drawn to the ventral surface of the embryo as, concurrently with lateral folding, the earliest heart tubes are drawn to meet at the midline, where they fuse together to form a single tubular heart that then complexly spiralizes. Meanwhile, islands of blood have started to coalesce in the yolk sac and then the body of the embryo to form vessels that will ramify with the developing heart. By 3 weeks the primitive heart is beating so it is generally recognized as the first organ system to reach a functional state.

Arteries are strong tubular structures that contain a pressurized fluid, the blood; they are formed of another tissue that is largely mesodermal in origin. All arteries have a smooth muscle layer that is usually circular but can, in the vastness of the arterial tree (which could be compared to one side of the world's road network), spiralize or assume a longitudinal banding depending on local hemodynamic. Because arteries are both intrinsically strong and pressurized, the blood vessels are a major constraining factor in growth (Blechschmidt & Gasser 1978), as at this early stage of embryogenesis the stiffer structures are the notochord and the arteries. Stiff arteries will tend to flex the body as the vertebrate body-plan features a cardiovascular system placed ventral to the gut tube. The arms and legs probably flex at the elbows and knees because of the relative shortness of the ventral arteries.

The pulsatile domain of the C-CF needs to be considered when contemplating disorders of movement. With the advent of the sphygmomanometer, blood pressure has become (along with temperature) one of the most measured physiological parameters. Hypertension is now recognized as being very widely spread amongst the world's population with figures quoted of up to 1.5 billion people afflicted. Complications of this silent killer are stroke, congestive heart disease, heart attacks, kidney damage or failure, arterial hardening, dementia, and eye disease.

To counter this almost systemic world disease, exercise needs to be increased, diets improved, salt and sugar intakes reduced, and alcohol intake moderated. It is a multifactorial disease of lifestyle so lifestyle changes are in order.

As suggested in Chapter 11, I recommend a revaluing of a floor-based lifestyle as one of the changes that can make a difference. Floor living encourages normal movement patterns across the biggest joints and muscles of the body. The arterial and venous tree has co-evolved with the needs imposed on it by bipedalism, but also it has evolved around resting shapes that are common to all humankind. I suggest sitting in a chair to rest after exercise is not as congruent with efficient hemodynamics as floor sitting. The vertical height from foot to heart that blood has to rise is considerably increased when chair sitting. Giraffes, for example, have evolved a blood pressure that is two times the large mammalian norm so that there is adequate arterial pressure to reach the raised head. Imagine blowing up a 5 cm straw or a 5 m straw to gain a sense of the importance of height to blood pressure. Habitual floor sitting should help especially as floor sitting is coupled with erecting from the floor, a subject I will also discuss in the next section.

Lifting weights, be it external weights or body weight, raises blood pressure. An experienced weightlifter during a double-leg press was recorded as having a blood pressure in excess of 480/350 mmHG (MacDougall et al 1985). The same study recorded mouth pressures of 30–50 Torr during a single maximum lift. A colleague, Phillip Silverman, is a weightlifter. During a heavy squat he reports that one of the primary feelings is that of extreme pressure in his head. When students on his Exercise Science course ask him what muscles he is using he replies, 'What muscles aren't I using?' Modelling movement without conceptually encompassing the pulsatile and the pulmonary/peristaltic systems is just inadequate. Without the enormous bracing that this transient spike in blood pressure must give to the body it would be impossible to lift that weight. Blood and visceral muscle are as mesodermal as the quadriceps and the erector spinae. This extreme example illustrates the essential need for a blood pressure response to a musculoskeletal load. I suggest rising from the floor 50–100 times a day will help self-regulate blood pressure, as will the regular lifting of light to moderate weights. Ally these lifestyle changes with wholefoods that are low in salts and hydrogenated fats so that the CVS may be functionally enhanced.

Cardiovascular health is essential to the moving body. When the case history or clinical examination points to blood pressure abnormalities, they must be factored in as contributing to the presenting musculoskeletal distress.

THE PERISTALTIC C-CF

For the purposes of this model the gastrointestinal tract and the muscle of the bronchial tree will be considered as one and called the peristaltic domain of the C-CF. The adult intestinal canal is about 8.0 m long with longitudinal and circular muscles. These muscles and associated structural tissues are derived from the splanchnic leaf of mesoderm that lies deep to the coelom.

Peristalsis is a wave-like motion that moves food from mouth to anus. Peristaltic movement is in response to a swelling within the lumen of the intestine that causes it to contract the lumen just proximal to the bolus of food, whilst just distal to the bolus, the lumen wall is relaxed. Remarkably, this muscular action is driven by a disseminated nerve plexus within the intestine so that, even if all the extrinsic nerves are cut to the intestine, the peristaltic movement continues in response to a local swelling within the intestine (Gershon 1998). The tone of this collectively vast muscle influences average transit times.

Paul Chek, at a seminar in the UK in 2002, described a training session with his son. That morning they measured their ability to hollow the abdomen via a blood pressure cuff. Lunch was a hot chilli dish. That afternoon when they returned to a training session they were both unable to generate the same abdominal hollowing, presumably because the chilli had inflamed their gut tube, a discomfort that they could both feel. The muscles of the abdominal wall will not be able to contract efficiently when there is visceral inflammation.

When the transit times are too rapid, the intestines will carry less food product and so offer less bracing for the exterior muscles to act about. If there are slow transit times, the intestine will carry more food product within that will create a relative stiffening of the intestinal motility. The intrinsic and extrinsic movements of the small intestine and large bowel will be compromised, in turn affecting the nuanced movement of the abdominal wall muscles that overlie the viscera. For optimal whole-organism movement the GIT needs to be able to writhe freely within its normal range of movement, uninhibited by tethering from scars, abdominal masses, and inflammation.

Research that explores movement solely with reference to the musculature of the external body wall and limbs will not approximate what the human physique is capable of. We need to develop models that incorporate blood pressure and the overall tonus or viscosity of the abdominal contents if we are to understand what we see athletes are actually capable of.

REFERENCES

Blechschmidt E, Gasser R 1978 Biokinetics and biodynamics of human differentiation. Thomas, Illinois

Gershon M 1998 The second brain. Harper Perennial, New York

Larsen W 1993 Human embryology. Churchill Livingstone, New York

MacDougall J, Tuxen D, Sale D et al 1985 Arterial blood pressure response to heavy resistance exercise. Journal of Applied Physiology 58(3):785–790

McManus C 2002 Right hand, left hand. Phoenix, London

NASA Astrobiology Institute. Could life be based on silicon rather than carbon? Available: http://nai.arc.nasa.gov/astrobio/feat_questions/silicon_life.cfm 15 June 2009

Fluid field (F-F)

10

Fluids enable all physiology. All movement is ultimately derived from fluid movement. As Novalis (1772–1801) of the early German Romantic movement noted, 'There is no doubt that our body is a moulded river.'

A modelling process develops its own inertia as the primary building blocks that have been selected for the model interact to approximate the system being modelled. As insight is generated via the model it then suggests new avenues for exploration. A fluid field (F-F) is postulated for two reasons.

Firstly, the embryology of mesoderm suggests the need for this field. The mesoderm used by the embryo to construct muscles and bones, both of the body-wall and the contractile elements of the viscera, also creates a visceral organ – the two kidneys that are derived from the intermediate mesoderm. At first glance it has always struck me as anomalous that mesoderm had this investment in the kidneys. All the derivatives of mesoderm introduced so far seemed to support or propel some part of the body whereas the kidneys sit well tethered by fascia and blood vessels behind the peritoneum where they filter fluid extruded from arterial blood vessels. What role might the kidneys play in the mesodermal world of movement?

Secondly, there is a more theoretical, almost metaphysical need for this field. At present our best bet for finding life in the universe is to look for water. All known animal life is essentially compartmentalized fluid water that is somehow animated. The CF model needed to create a space where fluid biodynamics hold center court. As the Chinese say, 'the Kidneys are the water viscus; they govern fluids and humour' (Flaws 1994), or more recently the sinologists Claude Larre and Elisabeth Rochat de la Vallée (Larre & Vallée 1999) when discussing the Kidneys state, 'The Kidneys represent the origin of life and the ability of life to reproduce exactly from the original model of life. They are the guarantee and the keeper of the pattern of life, in the same way that there must be a pattern for the knitting. At the level of the kidneys, essences are most faithful to themselves and to oneself. They are used to make another life with their richness and power. These are the essences for the reproduction of life, essences of sexuality.' Traditional Chinese Medicine

125

DOI: 10.1016/B978-0-7020-3109-0.00015-8

(TCM) has for millennia given great importance to the kidneys, far more than their small size and tucked away location should suggest to a pre-scientific medical community.

The F-F takes a wide-angle view of the primary fluid systems found in the mammalian body. These fluids include the cerebrospinal fluid, the remnants of the coelomic fluids, the vast interstitial fluid, the lymphatic fluid, the urinal fluid, the synovial fluids, sweat, seminal fluid, and milk. Blood, another fluid that is largely of mesodermal origin, is modelled within the pulsatile aspect of the chiralic CF, but the fluid aspect of blood, the plasma, is closely physiologically coupled to interstitial fluid, that ubiquitous fluid that surrounds the billions of cells that collaborate to form the body. If any of these fluids is under or over produced, or blocked in its normal physiological movement, expect consequences, often severe, in whole-organism movement patterns.

Early in embryogenesis these fluids are less compartmentalized so it is possible to consider a commonality of fluids that interact via the kidney. Unlike the other contractile fields this field is modelled as being non-contractile but nevertheless provides the basis for all movement of the body.

EVOLUTIONARY PERSPECTIVE

Metabolism produces by-products that must be eliminated from the body. Many of these metabolic by-products are water soluble, or are rendered water soluble, so the internal environment of the vertebrate has developed organs to meet the dual challenges of the excretion of the unwanted products of metabolism, whilst maintaining a water/salt balance. The excretory system of the vertebrate body includes the kidneys, the skin, gills and/or lungs, and specialized salt-excreting or salt-absorbing structures. (Note that in this context the large intestine expels the undigested products of digestion but only the bile fluids are excreted as such.) Vertebrate excretory systems have adapted to cope with both sea- and freshwater, or a terrestrial environment that can be water-rich or extremely desiccating. Because of the diverse challenges faced by the internal milieu the kidney system reflects its long convoluted evolutionary history via a developmental complexity that has fascinated biologists for well over 100 years.

The vertebrate kidneys have evolved because, unlike most invertebrates that are isotonic (equal in osmotic concentration) to seawater, most vertebrates, both aquatic and terrestrial, are hypotonic (lower in osmotic concentration) to seawater, but hypertonic (higher in osmotic concentration) to freshwater. Marine bony fishes constantly lose water by osmosis to the surroundings because the salt content of their bodily fluids is less than that of the seawater (hypotonic). To counter this net water loss, bony fish pass little urine as their renal corpuscles are small and poorly vascularized (Hildebrand 1982). Also they drink copiously but actively expel salt via the gills. Some sharks, marine reptiles, and birds that eat salty food have developed salt glands that collect, concentrate, and then expel the excess salt.

In contrast, freshwater fish are hypertonic to freshwater so they will tend to absorb water through any diffusible surface (gills, gut lining, skin) from the environment. To counter this net water influx their kidneys are specialized to produce copious but dilute urine; additionally, they can secrete mucus to cover diffusible surfaces, and they drink very little. Osmoregulation is absolutely vital but it requires the expenditure of considerable energy to maintain the composition of the interstitial fluids within narrow parameters via the elimination or conservation of water and salts (Liem et al 2001).

Amphibians, by definition, spend time on land so they must conserve water. Their kidneys are based on their freshwater ancestors so they can produce copious urine, some of which can be reabsorbed from the bladder to prevent loss. Another site of water loss is their thin skin that can act as a respiratory membrane. To counter this water loss, amphibians tend to prefer moist habitats where they can frequently return to the water to rehydrate.

Fully terrestrial lives needed physiologies better suited to water conservation, allied with an ability to convert waste nitrogen into urea that is chemically inert and requires little water for its removal. Mammals compound these physiological challenges as they are physically active and maintain their body temperature despite changes in ambient temperature, both of which use and lose yet more water. Mammals have met these challenges in large part by developing a unique kidney.

Some primitive vertebrates have only one pair of nephrons (the structural and functional unit of the kidney) per body segment; that number can rise to 3 or 4 million for the permanent human kidneys. Filtration pressure via arterial blood pressure has massively increased, so much so that about 25% of cardiac output is directed to the kidneys. The mammalian kidney also employs an evolutionary innovation called a countercurrent multiplier mechanism that acts on a new architecture of the nephron called the loops of Henle. The microcirculation of the kidney employs a high-pressure capillary network juxtaposed with a low-pressure capillary network that surrounds the loops of Henle. The enormous surface area for filtration, combined with the closely juxtaposed arterio-venous network, is able to process 180 liters of fluid per day, which is about ten complete sweeps of the body's entire extracellular fluid. Of the 180 liters, about 99% is returned via the loops of Henle to the extracellular fluid, with only 1 or 2 liters lost per day as urine (Despopoulos & Silbernagl 1986).

EMBRYOLOGICAL PERSPECTIVE

The embryology of the kidneys reflects their convoluted evolutionary history. Three sets of 'kidneys' develop in mammalian embryos: the pronephros and the mesonephros, which are transient embryonic kidneys that reflect the evolutionary development of the organ, and the metanephros from which the permanent kidney of the mammalian adult will develop. They all originate in a cephalic to caudal sequence from a ridge of intermediate mesoderm between the somites and the lateral plates (that lie on either side of the coelom and contribute to the body-wall and the muscles of the viscera). From this intermediate position the kidney precursors transitorily span from the lower cervicals all the way down to the sacral region. Intermediate mesoderm also contributes to the formation of the genital system so the two are commonly described as the urogenital system.

The pronephros is the first aspect of the embryonic kidney to manifest. It differentiates from the anterior pole of the intermediate ridge as a few renal tubules that open into the coelom that at this stage arcs over the cardiac region (day 25). It is functionally important to some fish species but in mammals it is a transient structure of mesodermal origin that has entirely disintegrated by the fourth week. Of interest here is the relationship between the pronephros and the coelom.

The primitive vertebrate kidney was segmented in a similar way to the somite segments of the spinal region, with each kidney segment placed between the coelom (which the kidney segment may open to) and the plasma fluids driven from the artery that emerged from that somitic segment. So urine is produced by these primitive kidney nephrons that accessed fluids from the coelom and the blood. Urine is drained via a longitudinal tube that formed by joining all the kidney segments to terminate in the cloaca (the 'sewer,' a common termination of the gut tube and the embryonic urogenital region).

Before the coelom compartmentalizes it is a horseshoe-shaped structure that opens to the outside of the embryo via two canals. At this stage many fluid systems are interconnected, all filtered by the embryonic kidneys and the placental circulation.

As the pronephros degenerates the next stage of kidney development produces the mesonephros, the middle kidney. The mesonephros is a bilateral elongated ovoid-like organ of about 70–80 tubules (in total) that lose contact with the coelom but drain their urine into the tube that was first established by the pronephros; this tube is so well described by Casper Wolff (1733–1794)

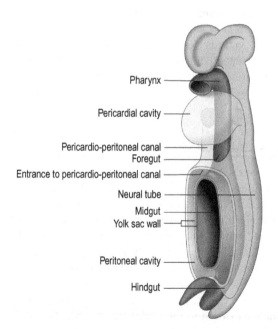

Pharynx

Pericardial cavity

Pericardio-peritoneal canal
Foregut
Entrance to pericardio-peritoneal canal
Neural tube
Midgut
Yolk sac wall

Peritoneal cavity

Hindgut

FIG 10.1 **Fluids of the body share a commonality that transcends locality** In early embryonic development the coelom is a primary conduit for fluid interchange between intra-embryonic and extra-embryonic fluids. *Adapted from Standring 2008.*

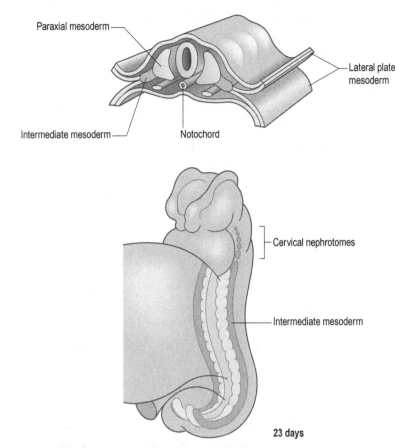

FIG 10.2 The intermediate mesoderm gives rise to paired, segmentally organized nephrotomes from the cervical to the sacral region. *Adapted from Larsen 1993.*

that it is commonly called the Wolffian duct (as distinct from the Wolffian ridge). Both the pronephros and the mesonephros produce a hypotonic urine (Williams 1995) that suggests these primitive organs of excretion evolved in a freshwater environment, but the story is typically bio-complex (see Wake 1979 and Liem et al 2001 for more detail). As this kidney stage degenerates the tube to the cloaca is appropriated by the developing male genital system to become the vas deferens.

The metanephros or permanent kidney is the third and final stage of the urine-producing organs. Two buds sprout from the caudal end of the Wolffian duct near the cloaca. These ureteric buds will elongate to form the left and right ureters, and induce the intermediate mesoderm in the region of the sacrum to form the permanent kidneys. In contrast to the pronephros and the mesonephros the metanephros produces a hypertonic urine. From a sacral origin the metanephros ascends to the level of the second lumbar vertebra.

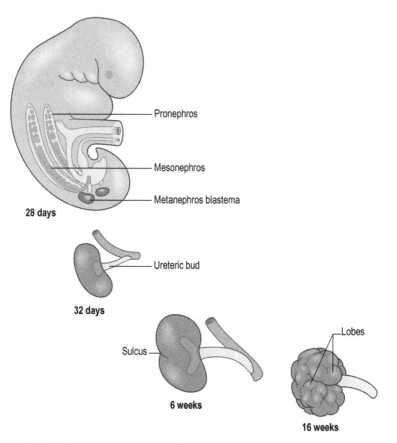

FIG 10.3 The origin of the permanent kidney – the metanephric kidney early in the 5th week Note that it develops its own drainage duct that will become the ureter. The defunct mesonephric duct is appropriated by the developing male gonads to become the vas deferens. *Adapted from Larsen 1993.*

THE FLUID FIELD

The two kidneys are placed on the dorsal surface of the internal body-wall at the level of T12, L1, L2, and L3, with the right kidney being about 2 cm lower than the left. With the ribs above and the ilia below, this region of the spine is subject to torsional biodynamics when we walk, run, and throw. When we want to remove water from a wet towel we do not pull or squeeze it, rather we contra-twist it. Are the kidneys able to exploit their position to help their physiology?

There is a commonality to all the fluids of the body. The common organs of excretion and osmoregulation for all fluids are the kidneys. The F-F is not contractile per se but as everything is sheathed in fascia, everything is susceptible to changes in fluid tonicity. The F-F is an attempt to recognize the centrality of fluid dynamics to life, and hence movement, via a model that places the kidneys as intermediate to the spinal structures behind and the structures of the lateral plate mesoderm. I have come to associate intermediate biodynamics with helical, writhing, twisting movements, which are the flow patterns preferred by fluids (Schwenk 1965).

In the clinical setting, simple advice concerning fluid physiology will help our movement-impaired patients. Advise them to: take much less salt and sugar, drink plain water rather than sugared drinks, moderate alcohol intake, sweat regularly, and walk/run for 45 minutes per day to counter-twist the waist region. Mesodermal kidneys need exercise, as do all the other mesodermal structures.

REFERENCES

Despopoulos A, Silbernagl S 1986 Color atlas of physiology. Georg Thieme Verlag, Stuttgart

Flaws B 1994 Statements of fact in Traditional Chinese Medicine. Blue Poppy Press, Boulder, CO

Hildebrand M 1982 Analysis of vertebrate structure, 2nd edn. John Wiley, New York

Larre C, Rochat de la Vallée E 1999 Essence, spirit, blood and Qi. Monkey Press, London

Larsen W 1993 Human embryology. Churchill Livingstone, New York

Liem K, Bemis W, Walker W, Grande L 2001 Functional anatomy of the vertebrates. An Evolutionary Perspective, 3rd edn. Harcourt College Publishers, Fort Worth

Schwenk T 1965 Sensitive chaos; the creation of flowing forms in water and air. Rudolf Steiner Press, London

Standring S 2008 Gray's anatomy, 40th edn. Churchill Livingstone, Philadelphia

Wake M 1979 Hyman's comparative vertebrate anatomy, 3rd edn. University of Chicago Press, Chicago

Williams P 1995 Gray's anatomy, 38th edn. Churchill Livingstone, Edinburgh

Archetypal postures

A self-tuning mechanism

Contractile fields are whole-organism in scope. We now need to develop a whole-organism approach to assessing musculoskeletal tune, i.e. the patterns of shape that emerge from the interaction of the contractile fields. The archetypal postures are appropriate as they are evident in our evolutionary history, our embryological/childhood development, and in our daily life, that is, until recently. Then we stopped using these postures to settle into chairs and sofas. The price has been musculoskeletal distress.

Back pain is endemic in our modern lives. This debilitating condition often proves resistant to understanding and treatment (Deyo 1993). What are the common denominators for this near universal dis-ease?

As a species we have a history that is at least 6 million years old. Some apes acquired a bipedal stance and our lineage developed this new gait by fine-tuning our musculoskeletal structure to walk and run in a biomechanically efficient way. Every single joint and muscle we have reflects this ancestry. After all, we are derived from *Homo erectus* – ancestral men and women who stood erect. However, preceding walking and running, both during our evolutionary development and our own childhood development, we first lie and then sit on the floor, and only then begin to erect ourselves from the floor.

133

© 2010 Elsevier Ltd / Inc / Bv
DOI: 10.1016/B978-0-7020-3109-0.00016-X

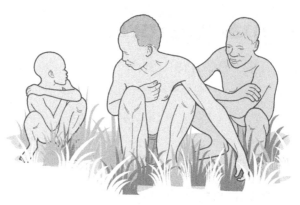

FIG 11.1 Floor living, rough terrain for the feet, and resource transport are the evolutionary heritage of our musculoskeletal system.

A whole-organism approach to musculoskeletal anatomy and function will both require and facilitate a new approach toward assessment. Contractile fields (CFs) model human movement. The opposite of human movement is human rest – movement and rest are flip sides of the same coin. One without the other is nonsensical. The key point here is the deep relationship between our movement patterns and our rest patterns, specifically the morphology of rest. I propose terrestrial animal bodies have evolved to be self-tuning via the regular use of postures of repose. Biomechanical tune is a vitally important concept that is hard to even consider from the perspective of structural anatomy – it would be like considering how to tune a car engine by looking at a piston. When anatomy is based on dismembering a body (as is structural anatomy) it is hard to see the living whole that is intrinsically grounded in relationship.

This book suggests we can reduce the incidence of musculoskeletal distress effectively and cheaply via three simple understandings.

Firstly, we, as a society, need to spend more time on the floor. All humans, all cultures, all ages have, until recently, spent all our resting and much of our working lives on the ground. Humans have two primary floor sitting postures, with many variations on the two. In the first series of postures we squat, long sit, or sit Japanese style (kneel). In the second primary style of floor sitting we turn our legs to side-sit or sit cross-legged (this primary group has the legs internally or externally rotated). It is proposed that these 'archetypal postures of repose' are a self-tuning mechanism for our complex musculoskeletal system. All big systems (and we are a big system) develop self-corrective capacities to preserve harmony between the many hierarchical levels of the system. Removing self-corrective modes is asking for trouble. We need floor sitting to preserve our biomechanical tune that is the profound interaction of many muscles and joints that summate to produce floor postures that provide us with ease and rest. I will develop these themes of 'tune' and archetypal postures later in this chapter.

Secondly, we then need to stand erect from sitting, an idea and exercise system I call *erectorcise*. Think about our modern lives. All of us spend our first years fighting gravity to learn to sit, and then to stand. It is a primordial anti-gravity urge. As adults we will lose that urge to fight gravity if we do not exercise these deeply embedded neuromuscular patterns. Our society is neglecting this crucial suite of movement patterns.

In the morning we get out of bed, but the bed is raised up to chair height so we do not put our musculoskeletal system through a full range of movement as we first stand. We then stagger to the toilet, again at chair height. Breakfast is sitting or standing, getting to work is sitting or standing, whilst work for many is prolonged chair sitting. On a good day we will go to the gym but many of the exercises are based on machines that are often constructed so that we sit to exercise. After sitting or standing we get home to once again sit for dinner, followed by a sofa for television. Many adults rarely do a full transition from the floor to standing.

Erecting ourselves from the floor is an essential tonic exercise that is a direct challenge to gravity. To stand up from the floor requires hundreds of muscles to work in complex choreography to take many kilos from the floor upward. And we would all have done this many times a day, every day, from the day we discovered how to stand erect, all the way through our lives, until we finally resign ourselves to bed and bedpans. If you want to preserve your mobility, and the mobility of your clients, start with simple exercises that involve the floor to standing transition.

Thirdly, our feet need functional rehabilitation. Feet to a biped are very special. Instead of four limbs we need to do the same duties with two. All big systems run on information. Feedback and feedforward are essential loops that inform and regulate a system. Feet are as biologically important as the eyes, ears, nose, hands, nipples, and genitals, as all are embryologically linked via the Wolffian ridge. To cover the feet with thick rubber is to specifically, but detrimentally, target the low back by reducing feedback and feedforward loops.

All day I listen to people describing their low back pain. From a biomechanical perspective our species has real vulnerability in the low back region. Contributing factors include our erect posture that places much more weight on the lumbar spine and the intervening intervertebral discs (IVDs). In addition we have made a pact with the biomechanical devil by utilizing the H-CF for our gait and throwing patterns as, paradoxically, our lumbar IVDs are particularly vulnerable to twisting insults.

Each spinal segment has an army of muscles that start at that level and course downward. Each spinal segment issues a pair of nerves that control the muscles starting from that segment, and supply a segmentally related patch of skin. The most vulnerable spinal segments are found at the junctional area of the lumbar spine and the sacrum (L4/L5 and S1), which send their sensory spinal nerves down to the sole of the foot, i.e. the most vulnerable segments are driven by the most information. This is important. The small muscles of the low back are thus segmentally related to the soles of the feet. Information drives all systems so here we have a sensory platform devoted to the most vulnerable region of the low back. Shoes, from this perspective, are sensory deprivation chambers that cut down the raw information we need to stand and walk in our precarious upright manner. To counter this I suggest to my patients they take their shoes off and walk barefoot on rough ground.

As that is often not possible in a city strewn with broken glass, the way to go is to build a rock garden for your home or office. I estimate our feet need about 20 minutes a day on a rough surface to keep our balance, our antigravity and our low spine muscles in good shape. A rock garden is easy to build, will soon be enjoyable, and will help retain good balance and reduce musculoskeletal pains.

Each of these topics will now be addressed in more detail. We will start with the concept of tune.

BIOMECHANICAL TUNE

We all have the sense of being 'in-tune' or 'out-of-tune.' Tune in the sense used here refers to hundreds of muscles and joints interacting in such a way that internal biomechanical friction and dissonance are kept to a minimum. Necessarily, the appreciation of biomechanical tune will involve a sense of aesthetics in the domains of human shape and movement. It is a sense that is at once obvious to most adults, and yet can be enhanced to a considerable extent. For example, if you were unfamiliar with hatha yoga or tai chi chuan but went to watch a class you would quickly appreciate the more advanced practitioners of those arts. Their movement would exude a power and poise that those less skilled would not. As your appreciation of these arts deepened your insight into the generation of that power and poise would develop. Subtle attention to good form combined with the nuanced placing and transfer of weight would become apparent. I am reminded of the long, black, pleated, skirt-like trousers used in aikido, which are designed to hide just this type of information from the non-initiated. Watching any sport is pleasurable because an appreciation of good form seems to transcend the hubris of daily life.

In many physiological domains, tune is already quantifiable. For example, a physical check-up with your doctor will involve height, weight, and waist relationships, your blood pressure, and key blood parameters. All are referenced to norms that have emerged from the study of many thousands of healthy folk. These physiological norms represent, and emerge from, the harmonious interaction of many physiological variables at lower levels of the biological hierarchy. Blood pressure emerges from heart and kidney function, these organs interacting with genes, diet, fitness levels, emotional state, and so on. But from all those sublevels emerge norms that can be assessed. The concept of tune from a CF perspective can be assessed via archetypal postures of repose.

Tune is not optional – it is the whole point to emergent systems.

As an analogy, suppose a musician is about to go on stage and the assistant offers two instruments – one is a hand-made work of art but it is out of tune, the other is old, battered and was always cheap, but this instrument is in tune. The musician has no choice but to take the instrument that is in tune. Tune emerges from the whole instrument, adjusted to criteria, often aesthetic, that harmoniously blend together many variables. A tuned instrument transcends itself – it is ready for music.

Lying and sitting on the floor have preceded human movement throughout our evolutionary development. Our bodies are profoundly configured to rest, to be at ease, on the floor. Chairs have introduced a new way of life that prevents us from assuming archetypal postures that all people, all ages, and all cultures have used for rest, recuperation, and I suggest, the re-tuning of our musculoskeletal system back to deeply embedded morphological norms.

In my practice I now see more young people suffering from being out of tune. Here is a possible scenario. Most Western children have bicycles. Humans have had 6 million years to embody floor postures, walking, and running. We have had 150 years to adapt our legs to bicycle cranks that move in a perfect circle. A group of muscles is drawn from a matrix to turn the crank. When the child gets home, slouching on chairs or sofas is the norm. Muscle tissue that is hot and pliable now cools whilst sitting on a chair. If you keep a chair posture without the chair being there to support you it is a posture of maximum exertion for the quadriceps group. Ten minutes in that posture will cause extreme fatigue, shaking and pain. When sitting in a chair, hot, vasodilated muscle cools and sets like jelly – setting in a shape that the body associates with maximum exertion. The effect is compounded in children as their anterior pituitary gland releases growth hormone so muscle is additionally stretched by bone growth. Relationships between major muscle compartments in the leg become subtly deranged. Joints act as hard mediators between these compartments so they become stressed. Joint capsules (the ligamentous collar that joins one bone to another) become too loose or too tight, with attendant vulnerabilities such as joint instabilities and chronic compressions.

Every day in practice I see evidence of musculoskeletal systems that are out of tune. I have noticed, for example, that knee joint crepitus (the crackling noise associated with joint movement) is directly associated with loss of ease in the archetypal postures. Many adults will produce a distressing noise from their knees when they try to fully squat but babies do not have noisy joints. When you cannot fully squat (knees over second toe, heels down, arches lifted), the knee intra-compartmental pressures are malignly altered so that wear and tear in the joint is accelerated. I have heard crepitus from the knee joints of a 15-year-old, a teenager who was otherwise fit and healthy. Over years, being out of tune will gradually distort your musculoskeletal structure and lead to premature aging of the legs and low back in particular. It is no accident that it is our culture that has invented hip and knee replacements. Because the body's musculature is so networked, when the legs and low back are in distress they tend to set up satellite distress in the neck and shoulders. The CF model helps to track how that distress will permeate and manifest around the body. Many areas of pain manifest, each with a named diagnosis, but most of this distress is emanating from a common cause.

Tuning your musculoskeletal system via archetypal postures of repose, strengthening your body's ability to erect itself from the floor, and rehabilitating your feet, will turn on powerful self-corrective modalities.

A SELF-TUNING MECHANISM

Archetypal postures of repose are simple postures that benefit the musculoskeletal system. The disturbingly simple take-home message is to re-value the floor by sitting on it. That is all that is required. Floor-based living does not ask for your time, nor are there any particular exercises you need do. It is a concept that is easy to impart to your patients, a concept that is deceptively simple and obvious, but profound in its effects on musculoskeletal function.

> Before I begin to describe the postures, the usual caveats apply. If you have had joint replacements or reconstructions these postures may well be outside your new range of movement. Do not attempt them without advice from your orthopedic surgeon. Following vascular surgery you will also need advice from your surgeon. Be very careful getting up and down from the floor if you have lost access to this primal movement pattern. Have a friend on hand to help you up if need be.

I will describe ways of getting down to and erecting from the floor that will minimize the chance of hurting yourself. Beware of slippery surfaces and rugs that may move from under you. Do not spend too much time in any one posture. Move with care from one posture to another as you feel the need. Gradually increase the time you are able to spend on the floor. Imagine yourself as a bonsai tree that has grown with a displeasing aesthetic. The errant branches must be reshaped slowly, so too we must allow time for ease to re-emerge. Change shape slowly via comfortable but prolonged stretches (Light et al 1984). Gently ease yourself toward tune, particularly if you are strong but stiff, older, arthritic, or very overweight.

Archetypal postures are essential after exercise. The usual post-exercise stretching appears to be a waste of time. Few studies find it helps with injury rates. I suggest it is the whole cool-down phase that is the important time period. To a hot, wet, vasodilated muscle that has just spent an hour running up a hill, a 30-second calf stretch is a rather insignificant task for the muscle. What is important is to sit on the floor in the various archetypal postures, thus re-establishing fundamental relationships between muscle compartments as they cool and set. After exercise go back to the floor as people, worldwide, have always done. Described below are the primary archetypal postures of repose, each of which has many subtle variants.

FULL SQUAT

The full squat is the quintessential human posture of repose. By way of introduction to this posture I recommend a book to you called *Lowly Origin: Where, When, and Why Our Ancestors First Stood Up* by Jonathan Kingdon (2003). Kingdon is both an artist and a world-renowned zoologist. His multivolume *East African Mammals: Atlas of Evolution in Africa* was voted in the Millennium issue of *American Scientist* magazine as one of the '100 books that shaped a century of science.' For decades, Kingdon has described the mammals of Africa and the environment in which they have evolved and now live. *Lowly Origin* takes that extraordinary cross-species perspective and turns it around to look at our species in a similar way. The book takes its title from a full squat as Kingdon has identified this posture as being essential to our evolutionary history. Squatting is a balance on two feet, what he calls a 'preadaptation' that facilitated a straight spine, allowed us to feed with two hands, and prepared us for bipedal standing. Squatting precedes standing: in a sense it is the sitting form of standing.

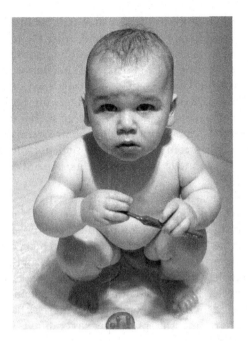

FIG 11.2   The full squat – a developmental birthright for all *Homo sapiens* Note the ease in the posture, and the relaxed upper body.

If a full squat was an essential piece in our evolutionary jigsaw it is also a key stage in our personal development. All babies squat, or if they do not they should be encouraged to do so by their parents and pediatric physiotherapist. At the anterior surface of the distal tibia, small squatting facets are frequently found. Squatting facets are more common in fetuses, Indian and Australian aboriginal populations, and pre-medieval European populations. They allow the deep dorsiflexion of the ankle needed in a barefoot full squat. Classical ballet, with its emphasis on pointing the foot, can cause the opposite of a squatting facet as an exostosis can develop that is a bony block to deep dorsiflexion, often causing impingement and pain. Our tendency to use heels on our shoes and to rarely assume this posture means many Western people find this a difficult posture to find ease in.

The ideal squat has the feet near parallel, the heels on the ground, and the knees over the second toe with no collapse of the medial arch of the feet. The tibialis anterior is relaxed as body weight has moved over the ankle's center of gravity. Pre-modern cultures would have found this posture an everyday fact of life. In New Zealand it tends to be cold and muddy so a full squat is frequently a more attractive option than a cross-legged posture that commits your sensitive bits to the terrain. The classic *Light on Yoga* by BKS Iyengar demonstrates hundreds of yoga postures, yet it does not have a photograph of a full squat, only difficult variations, like a full squat with a twist so that the hands interlock behind the back. It would seem that Iyengar did not think it was necessary to photograph a basic full squat because everyone was considered to be capable of assuming this posture; however, this is certainly not the case.

It is important to work toward this posture without hurting your knees or ankles. Many people attempting a full squat bring the knees medially and collapse on the medial arch of the feet. Squatting badly will just stress the knee and ankle inappropriately and make the situation worse. Start with the legs wider than the hips with the feet slightly turned out. Carefully squat down with the knees over the second toe, and let your heels come up. Hang onto a doorframe or something solid if you need to, but keep the shoulders down and back whilst they support the squat. Gradually the heels will descend as the Achilles complex lengthens and dorsiflexion of the ankle improves. Then start to move the feet to be more parallel and closer to the midline.

Ease in the full squat tunes the relationship between the muscles of the anterior and posterior compartments of the lower leg. Note that the anterior compartment (tibialis anterior, extensor hallucis longus, extensor digitorum longus, and peroneus tertius) is derived from the embryonic dorsal moiety, whereas the posterior compartment (gastrocnemius and soleus) is derived from the ventral moiety. Tuned dorsiflexion, as evidenced by a full squat, sets a relationship between dorsal and ventral that has a system-wide effect. When dorsiflexion is limited the anterior compartment muscles have to work against the stronger posterior compartment muscles so conditions such as shin splints are more likely to manifest.

The full squat is a full coiling of the leg's musculature. When the leg limb bud rotates and long axis twists, dorsal moiety muscle comes to lie on the ventral surface, and vice versa. If the full squat is limited, the coiling of the musculature is too tight. The half lotus posture described below is the uncoiling of the leg's musculature from this perspective.

In summary I suggest the full squat is a human posture of real importance to our biomechanical health, analogous to the middle C note on a piano. The squat is a posture used in primal activities such as labor and defecation. Many of my patients will never squat like a Kalahari bushman. Years of bicycles, high heels, and gym machines that isolate and train a muscle to exhaustion set relationships that will not be corrected easily. However, what is important is to claim back what you can of this posture as part of your floor repertoire. A small improvement in dorsiflexion is moving one toward tune. Ally that with a rock garden that helps bring the intrinsic muscles of the feet back to functionality and the therapeutic effects are surprisingly widespread.

TOE SITTING OR STANDBY POSTURE

From a squat it is easy (or should be) to move into the toe sitting posture. I also call this a standby posture, as the body is poised for movement. This is because the toes are extended in this posture so that the whole extensor pattern of the body is primed. In this posture the spine is upright, the toes are extended, and the knees rest on the floor. Most people find this a difficult posture to maintain, as the muscles and fascia of the sole of the foot are too tight to allow the metatarsal heads of the feet to fully rest on the floor. The toes do not fully extend and so they take too much body weight. If the posture is held and the toes become more painful the natural movement pattern is to use the quadriceps to sit up and raise the shoulders to lift away from the pain.

I have noticed how neck and shoulder pain is related to loss of ease in these archetypal sitting postures. Typically, patients present with an acute flare-up of a chronic pain in the neck and shoulder region. Frequently they say that the neck/shoulder region is the area where they hold their tension. In my experience, soft-tissue massage, stretching, spinal manipulation, and acupuncture do little to affect the deeper roots of this presentation. The treatment will usually help for a short time but invariably the chronic tension pattern returns. It is a whole-body loss of tune so just concentrating treatment on the presenting body part is likely to have a poor mid-term outcome. A similar pattern is seen in the full squat posture. When it is hard to squat comfortably (these are meant to be resting postures) the shoulders rise and hunch forward to bring body weight forward to make the squat easier. To help neck and shoulder distress I suggest local treatment in conjunction with advice regarding the archetypal postures to more fully address the dysfunctional pattern.

Frogs run their gastrocnemius muscle over the 'heel' and directly to the toes. Ease in the toe sitting posture normalizes deep relationships between the posterior compartment muscles of the calf, the plantar fascia, and the toes that are the sensitive end point of all the muscles of the leg. All the limb musculature expresses itself via the fingers and toes. In systems theory, you look for control points that are able to initiate or correct the system. Tuning the toes and feet is much more than just a local increase in flexibility.

Toe sitting can demonstrate another important insight associated with tune. When a musician is tuning an instrument they will test each note and listen for discordance. Likewise, in this musculoskeletal context, I look for discordance by palpating the body looking for trigger points. It is important to ask a 'normal question.' By this I mean a pressure that in my judgement, based on the size, weight, and health of the patient, should feel appropriate and good. The patient, asked a normal question of their musculoskeletal system, should respond normally.

When toe sitting, if the metatarsal heads are on the floor because the toes are fully extended, I find when I press the plantar fascia it usually feels good to the patient. When the toe sitting posture is difficult, the same pressure will cause a pain, analogous to a mal-tuned noise from an instrument. The patient will find a normal palpatory pressure on the arch of the foot painful. If I asked them to give a noise to the feeling it would be a noise of distress, or if I asked them for a color it would usually be a red or a color they associate with distress and pain. Trigger points start to become predictable in their location once the concept of normal tuned shape is grasped. Toe sitting is a normal posture for the human physique.

Ease into toe sitting by gradually spending more time in the posture, and by using a rock garden that I will describe later in the text. Take care if you have bunions, badly distorted feet, or a history of foot fractures and operations, etc. Even if the posture never becomes comfortable, moving toward ease is beneficial.

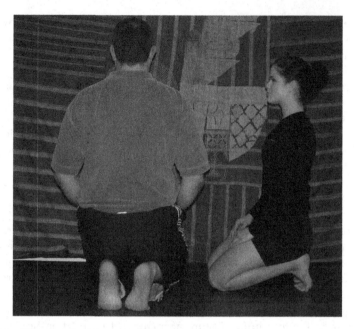

FIG 11.3 Sitting on the toes, a stand-by posture

THE DRINKING POSTURE

This is a posture that is similar to the toe sitting posture but, in this variation, the body is bent forward, forehead to the floor. I suggest this posture is archetypal because it is a posture that we would assume if, after a long desert crossing, we arrived at a river. The prayer posture is a drinking posture. The toes need to be extended otherwise one will tend to fall into the water.

From the toe sitting posture, bend forward with control toward the ground. Slightly contract the lower abdominal muscles and maintain control of the descent, using the hands on the ground to aid the descent of the forehead to the floor. When the body is in good tune it is possible to do this forehead-to-floor movement repeatedly without using the arms for support.

KNEELING

Here we have a floor posture that usually reminds people of Japanese culture. It is similar to toe sitting but has the dorsal surface of the foot on the ground, big toes usually just touching. In some cultures the feet may overlap so that the convex arch of one foot rests in the concave arch of the other foot. Many Western people find this a difficult posture to hold for any length of time. A traditional Japanese restaurant where one sits on tatami mats can cause enough discomfort to detract from the fine meal. However, it is a posture of rest as compared with the toe-sitting posture that is similar but with the toes extended so that the extensor fields are primed. When the quadriceps are too tight and the buttocks cannot rest on or between the heels it is indicative of an extensor pattern that is too primed. If you can sit comfortably in this posture, try lifting up a few centimeters and stay there for a few minutes. The

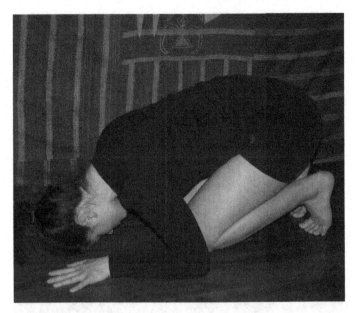

FIG 11.4   The drinking posture Extending the toes facilitates the ability to drink.

posture is very expensive on energy use – 5 minutes is very tiring and painful, getting to the point when you would willingly give your credit card details simply to get out of the position!

When the posture is difficult, use a pillow between the buttocks and the legs, and another between the ankles and the floor if need be. Using pillows and supports to make the archetypal postures easier is a necessary aid when the postures cause distress. Do not spend too long in the postures as it is important not to stretch the ligaments of the joints. Try to sit upright, shoulders down and back.

COWBOY POSTURE

The cowboy posture is a combination of a Japanese person sitting with one leg, whilst the other leg is up like a squat. It is a posture that is often assumed as a work posture as it is both stable and supportive for working in front of the body.

LONG SITTING

Long sitting is a common posture of repose in many parts of the world. Both legs are straight in front, with some cultures crossing one leg over the other just proximal to the ankle. To sit with a straight back in this posture is difficult if the hamstrings are too tight. If the low back is stressed in flexion by this posture it is better to slightly flex both knees to take the pressure off the low back.

Sitting in these postures builds a functional core strength as the abdominal wall is interacting with the powerful muscles of the hip joints.

143

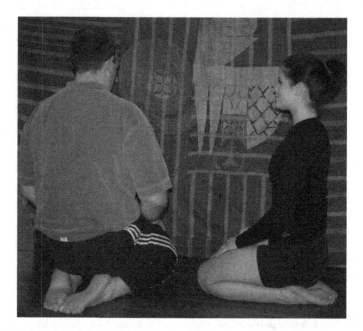

FIG 11.5   The kneeling posture

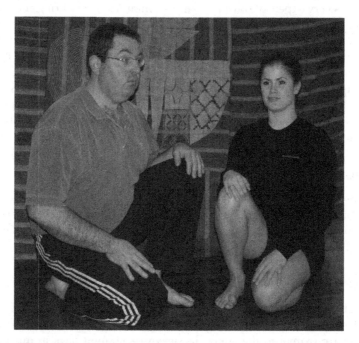

FIG 11.6   The cowboy posture

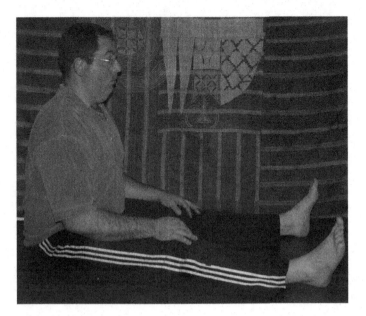

FIG 11.7 The long sitting posture

CROSS-LEGGED POSTURE

All the archetypal postures described above present the legs in a linear or straight manner. Conversely, the legs can be turned out at the hips and flexed at the knees to cross at the ankles. There are many variations on this posture. The legs may be tucked tightly one under the other, they can be crossed but not tucked under, or one foot may ride on the inner ankle of the other in a half-lotus posture.

People who find these cross-legged postures easy often do so because they are stiff in the more linear postures. Given a floor-sitting opportunity they will gravitate toward cross-legged rather than a Japanese posture or a squat. Ideally, one has access to both primary modes of sitting. In our Stone Age past the environment often dictated which posture was the most appropriate.

The half-lotus posture is a more advanced posture but I include it here as, in the past, the posture had its uses. If a thorn has penetrated the sole of the foot, turning it up to take a good look would have been normal procedure. Our contemporary life with our thickly wedged shoes means this is thankfully a rare event now but it is still biomechanically normal to be able to examine your upturned foot in this way. When the half-lotus posture becomes too difficult, people will struggle to get the foot up onto the contralateral inner thigh, and may do so by stressing the knee and the lateral ligaments of the ankle.

A sense of aesthetics in these postures is quickly taught. Students of mine have often contacted me months after a workshop to comment on their observations in clinical practice, and their own emerging ease in these postures.

145

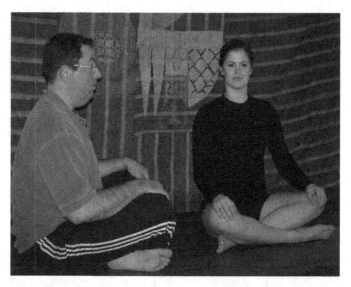

FIG 11.8 The cross-legged posture

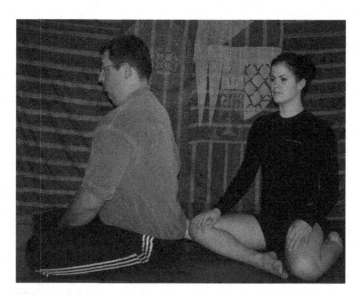

FIG 11.9 The side-saddle posture

SIDE-SADDLE POSTURE

Side-saddle posture refers to both legs to one or other side. One leg is externally rotated and the other is internally rotated. The lateral contractile field (L-CF) on the contralateral side to the legs is stretched. The posture is common amongst societies where it is inappropriate for women to sit with their legs apart.

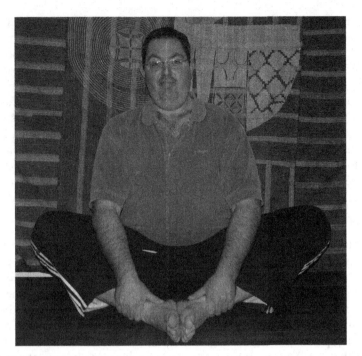

FIG 11.10   The tailor's posture

TAILOR'S POSTURE

This is another archetypal posture. Here one sits on the floor with the soles of the feet together in front of the pubis. Tailors of old assumed this posture whilst they held a fabric with their feet. However, the posture is far older than fabric. Neanderthal skeletons show wear marks on the incisor teeth where they held leather or plant material for plaiting, the other end being held by the feet in the tailor's posture, leaving both hands free for the job at hand.

The sartorius muscle is often associated with this posture as it externally rotates the leg and flexes the knee. After exercise, to sit in this posture and try to bend forward stretches groin tissue you did not know you had.

THE ERECTORCISE EXERCISES

From the floor, one must stand up. Erecting from the floor, also called a floor-to-standing transition, is a movement sequence that goes right to the heart of our human experience. We have all spent our early years training our musculoskeletal system to erect from the floor. The erectorcise exercises are derived from the many ways we can erect from the floor. If your musculoskeletal system will allow you to get down to the floor, these movement sequences are mandatory. They range from exercises that use supports to help one stand, all the way through to exercises that would be appropriate for elite athletes.

A forthcoming book will detail these exercises so here I will only introduce the exercise concept and talk about good technique as one arises from the floor. Like most people leading a modern city life, I too spend too much time in conventional chairs as our entire built world is predicated on chair sitting to work and rest. In contrast, if I spend an evening sitting on the floor I repeatedly find myself getting up and down from the floor: the door-bell rings, I have forgotten the cutlery, the phone rings, my glass is empty, etc. Over the course of a day, despite too much conventional sitting, I stand up from the floor between 50 and 100 times. The erectorcises are profoundly tonic to the largest muscles in your body, those muscles working in sequences that are embedded in the core design of our biomechanical structure.

ERECTORCISE BEGINNER

If you have not lived on the floor for many years, take care now to establish good form as you arise. Have a solid chair or table nearby, then from a cross-legged, floor sitting posture use your arms to help you twist up to a toe sitting posture. If the left leg is the outside leg, twisting to the right is usually the easiest way, and vice versa. Twisting on the way up and down from the floor is the most biomechanically efficient way of transitioning. Once you are in a toe sitting posture, bring one leg through so that the knee is over the second toe of that leg. You do not want to have the knee medial or lateral to the midline of the supporting foot. Now, to get up, push from the back toes that you have extended, help yourself with your arms if need be, and use the quadriceps group of the front leg to power up.

To erect from a Japanese sitting posture lift the buttocks to extend the hip joints, take one leg through to the front whilst concurrently extending the toes of the leg that is not taken forward. Push with the back toes as you lift using the leg you have taken forward, again using your arms to help if need be.

Getting down to the floor requires the same care. Do it step by step, respecting any pains you encounter. Holding onto a secure object, lower yourself to one knee then to the other so that you are again in the toe sitting posture, take one arm down to the floor by your side and descend to the floor. I suggest you spend a couple of weeks just getting up and down from the floor in daily life before moving to the next stage. Do remember these are postures that may have taken many years to lose access to so allow time for ease and strength to return. The Feldenkrais technique has explored some of these sequences in great depth.

ERECTORCISE INTERMEDIATE

You are comfortable on the floor in most of the archetypal postures. From here one can begin to train the erector muscles of the body by repeating floor-to-standing transitions with a variety of techniques and repetitions. Start with 10 times up/down as described above, 5 times with each leg; follow that with another 10 times getting up but now without the support of the secure object. Not using your arms makes a big difference. Then try 10 times from a supine lying posture to fully erect by rolling to a side and then twisting to a sitting position, to then stand erect. Another variation is to try 10 times rolling up or jumping up from a prone lying posture to fully erect. There are different ways of doing this – experiment and see what feels efficient for you. That is 40 repetitions of an archetypal push against gravity. Keep good form. If you get tired and form becomes disordered you must stop. Do not risk injury in the quest to tune and strengthen yourself.

ERECTORCISE ADVANCED

If you are in good form, strong and flexible, and at ease on the floor there are many ways of cranking these exercises up. From fully supine you can erect with no use of the twisting muscles. Bring your knees to your chest, roll on the back to build up momentum and go straight to a full squat and up. Repeat 10–40 times. From a full squat, erect 30–60 times. From a cross-legged posture bring your feet in tight with a little momentum and erect straight up, untwisting your legs as you stand. From a Japanese sitting posture explode up to a full squat, and then stand. There are many variations on a theme that will challenge most athletes.

Erectorcise exercises are a fundamental movement pattern that benefits everyone. They naturally emerge from floor living so decide now to eat your meals, listen to your music, and entertain your friends from the floor. If you also rehabilitate your feet, as I will describe next, you can expect significant improvements in your biomechanical well-being.

FREE YOUR FEET FROM THE SENSORY DEPRIVATION CHAMBERS

Feet are the organs we wedge into shoes before breakfast. All day they are constrained and sensorially isolated. When we eventually free them after we get home at night they are expected to negotiate carpets and flat floors, i.e. the lowest common denominator in that they experience no texture or balance needs. In my osteopathic practice I see some terrible feet. Think orthodontic dentist looking at a set of teeth that have been wearing a disastrous appliance for 40 years. Teeth (read foot bones) are pulled all over the place.

Shoes protect our feet but they have become far more than that. They have become fashion statements that subserviate the needs of the feet to our greater social ambition. Feet, sense organs of Wolffian ridge class, covered in leather and thick man-made cushioning, are reduced to a jumble of oversensitive, delicate and disordered tissue. This is polemical indeed but watching people walk across rough rocks at the seashore confirms the impression that most feet are far too dysfunctional and soft.

The lower lumbar and first sacral nerves innervate the skin of the sole of the foot and most of the intrinsic and extrinsic muscles of the foot are innervated from L4–S3. Nerves that innervate the foot are the same nerves that innervate the deep muscles of the pelvic floor and low back (such as the multifidus, the intertransversarii, the interspinales, and the rotatores lumborum). These small muscles act as vernier jets. A vernier jet is an auxiliary rocket engine that fine-tunes the attitude of a spacecraft. Short sharp blasts position the spacecraft in three dimensions. Like the fins of a fish, they need to be carefully placed to control the spacecraft's pitch, roll, and yaw. Used in this context the small low back muscles send short bursts of contractility amongst local vertebrae to fine-tune their positional relationships, one to the other.

The small deep muscles of the low back are designed to be the recipients of a massive stream of information in real time from the feet. Or rather they should be. Shoes dumb down the raw data the feet are capable of sending up to the low back. All systems need incoming data to self-regulate.

Even months after a painful low back episode, the multifidus muscles can carry a lingering deficit (Julie et al 1996). When intrinsic muscles of the spine are damaged the nervous system is able to re-route movement pathways around damaged tissue. Walking barefoot on rough ground challenges the intrinsic muscles of the low back to fully rehabilitate.

I suggest to some of my patients they build a 'rock garden' for their homes or workspace. A rock garden can be sized from 1 square meter to many square meters. I use thick plywood and bind stones of varying size and shape to the plywood using the glue that would join tiles to plywood. This type of glue sets like a solid rubber that is ideal for holding the stones. The stones are meant to be challenging to the feet so a real jumble of shapes and edges is OK. On my rock garden I have used red nail polish to mark out the stones that might hurt if they are stepped on too heavily. The rock garden needs to be in a place where it will be walked on for about 20 minutes per day. Kitchens, bathrooms, stairs, or walkways in the house or office would all be suitable. The rock garden certainly becomes a feature of the house!

Over a few months the results of this simple intervention to the life of your feet can be quite remarkable. As the intrinsic muscles of the feet come on-line the intrinsic muscles of the segmentally related low back are stimulated. Chronic back pains can diminish, balance will improve, shoulder tension will improve, and so on. It gradually becomes a pleasure to stand on a rock and massage the foot as one waits for the meal to cook.

SUMMARY

Back pain is a recurring distress for many people. We need new ways to think about its genesis and its treatment. Too much of the time we seem to be treating the consequences of a disordered musculoskeletal system rather than attending to some of the underlying issues that cause the disorder. I have suggested floor-based living is of real use to tuning the complex muscles of the waist, buttocks, and legs, toward deeply embedded functional norms. Erecting oneself from the floor is, likewise, a profound exercise. When this advice is allied to the rehabilitation of a major musculoskeletal organ – the feet – do expect a wide-ranging improvement in your well-being. Approaching back pain in this manner is not demanding of your time or your wallet. Manual therapy, in conjunction with this simple advice, can then aid rehabilitation in a meaningful manner.

WEBSITE

http://erectorcise.com/

REFERENCES

Deyo R 1993 Practice variations, treatment fads, rising disability. Do we need a new clinical research paradigm? Spine 18(15):2153–2162

Iyengar BKS 2001 Light on yoga. Thorsons, London

Julie A, Richardson C, Jull G 1996 Multifidus muscle recovery is not automatic after resolution of acute, first-episode low back pain. Spine 21(23):2763–2769

Kingdon J 1971–1982 East African mammals: atlas of evolution in Africa, 7 vols. University of Chicago Press, Chicago

Kingdon J 2003 Lowly origin: where, when, and why our ancestors first stood up. Princeton University Press, Princeton and Oxford

Light K, Nuzik S, Personius W, Barstrom A 1984 Low-load prolonged stretch vs. high-load brief stretch in treating knee contractures. Physical Therapy 64(3):330–333

Decoding the Chinese meridial map

12

> *We are consequently faced with the profoundly difficult problem of translating the medieval theories into terms of modern science, a process which may well prove impossible, yet traditional physicians used them for two and a half millennia for organising their vast clinical experience. There is a paradox here not yet resolved.*
> Lu & Needham 1980

In the late 1980s I decided to study Chinese acupuncture as I thought it would stretch my conceptual boundaries and be a valuable clinical adjunct to manual therapy. I learned that the practice of acupuncture within Traditional Chinese Medicine (TCM) is predicated on the existence of meridians (variously called channels, conduits, tracts, and Jinglùo). Meridians are lines on the surface of the body that did not seem to track any anatomical structure that I was aware of. The particular meridian might track with a muscle or a neurovascular bundle for some portion of its length, and then randomly diverge. Some meridians ran in straight lines, others zigzagged. At the time I can remember discussing what meridians might be with Carola

153

Beresford-Cooke, a respected shiatsu practitioner and author. Rather blandly I suggested the meridians might follow lines of fascia. As fascia ensheaths everything I was actually suggesting nothing. What did the Chinese map so confidently, so comprehensively, more than 2000 years ago?

The early Chinese medical theorists maintain they mapped the movement of Qi and Blood, a movement that was coalesced into a circuit of 12 meridians, with 2 more meridians mapping the dorsal and ventral midline. They saw the disturbance of Qi and Blood flow as being inherent to the genesis of disease. Early maps of meridians gave little precision to the lines and the acupoints. They appear to be more an aide-mémoire to be used in conjunction with personal tuition from a teacher. With the influence of Western medical practice in the early 1900s, meridian mapping became anatomically referenced. A modern text that I use as reference, *A Manual of Acupuncture* (Deadman et al 1998), runs to more than 600 pages of detailed anatomical description. Each meridian and the 360-odd acupoints have been mapped with reference to surface anatomy, direction, and depth of needling, and a commentary discussing historical and contemporary actions attributed to the acupoint. Other texts have explored the underlying cross-sectional anatomy beneath each acupoint (Jing 1982). There is a paradox here that I will come to.

Acupoints located on the meridians are needled in patterns called point prescriptions to treat disease. Typically, a clinical syndrome would be treated using 10–20 needles placed about the body and limbs so that the actions attributed to each acupoint summate and support each other to treat the syndrome. My osteopathic education was derived from a Western bioscientific perspective, so to learn that the Chinese treated shoulder conditions with needles to the lateral knee region, and headaches with needles inserted on the hands and feet, was then beyond my ability to comprehend. I had come to the subject wanting a conceptual stretch via a different cultural and historical paradigm, but I was also surprised by the amount of rote learning that was involved. As a student I would try to memorize this vast body of culturally encoded medical information by drawing small figurines, with each figurine depicting the symptoms and the acupoints used to treat that syndrome.

When I studied TCM and acupuncture in the late 1980s the meridial map was presented as an ancient, revered, and transmitted wisdom that was beyond our comprehension or questioning. One rote learnt, trusted the Chinese medical theorists knew what they where doing, and tried to pass exams. But there is a rub. Bioscience has looked in vain for the meticulously mapped meridians. Dissective studies, computerized axial tomography (CAT) scans, magnetic resonance imaging (MRI) scans, positron emission tomography (PET) scans, thermal imaging, radioactive tagging, scanning electron microscopy, and so on – the full armamentarium of modern medical investigative techniques has failed to demonstrate a physical substrate that is meridian-like. There are hints of something afield (such as endogenous opiates, skin rashes, some positive clinical outcomes, fascial winding from needles, etc.) but, to date, bioscience has been unable to fathom a contemporary understanding of the complex meridial map.

So here is the paradox: meridians are now described with meticulous reference to Western anatomy but anatomically they do not appear to

Muscles and meridians

exist. The situation is somewhat analogous to the use of herbs before pharmacology – herbs 'worked' but how they did so was unknown.

In the late 1990s, I was practicing and teaching osteopathy in London. I was working on the contractile field (CF) model of movement but it seemed that each additional insight took an inordinate amount of time and effort. I was reading embryology and trying to come to grips with limb development. One night I was looking at a scanning electron micrograph of a day 32 upper limb bud when I saw a similarity between the embryological description and the layout of the arm meridians. Embryologists described invisible lines on the center of the developing limb bud, and borders between the ventral and dorsal domains above and below the middle of the limb bud. The parallels I saw between the arcane lines of limb development and Chinese meridians kept me occupied for the next 6 months as I proceeded with a 'decoding' of the meridial map.

The map of meridians is the world's oldest medical map still in widespread clinical use. The practice of acupuncture is, in fact, now a global phenomenon with more than 2 billion people having access to this form of treatment. From a medical anthropological point of view the meridial map gives us access to some of the earliest recorded medical theory and practice. The Chinese give few clues to the genesis of the meridial map other than to say they mapped the *'movement of Qi and Blood.'* The word 'movement' I have come to think is the important part of the phrase as Qi (roughly translatable as life force) is too amorphous a concept, and the vessels it is supposed to travel in have never been identified. Similarly, a Western anatomical understanding of blood and the blood vessels it travels in bears no resemblance to the meridial map. So Qi and Blood seemed to offer few handles with which to start the attempt to see meaning in the meridial map. To decode the meridial map, to understand what was mapped, a better model of whole-organism movement was needed: this is where the CF model comes in.

RECOIL FROM PAIN

I suggest the Chinese did indeed map a form of movement, an obvious movement given the nature of needles and moxibustion (the burning of a herb near the skin). They mapped, in large part, 'recoil from a noxious stimulus.' When you are pricked or burnt (or pushed firmly with a finger) you will move coherently and quickly away from the source of hurt. Acupuncture as we know it today was predicated on the manufacture of suitable steel needles. Two thousand years ago, metallurgy in China could not produce the fine gauge, single use and disposable needles we now employ. A young acupuncturist 1500+ years ago would have saved for months to buy their leather roll of acupuncture needles, lances, and other instruments. That kit would have been used for a whole professional life. Acupuncture needles were made to last and they must have carried a real insertional sting with them.

Recoil as a neurological event has a history that dates back to the pre-Cambrian animal diversification. The earliest life on this planet (600+ MYA) was like the Garden of Eden in that there is little evidence of predation – life was tethered or floated randomly. The pre-Cambrian period ushered in an explosion of new animal body-plans, animals that moved volitionally with

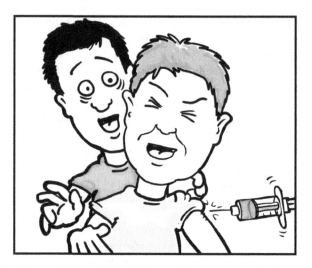

FIG 12.1 Recoil from pain has real survival value Acupuncture needles plug into that important reflex. *Original drawing by MONSTAcartoons (Mark O'Brien), © Elsevier.*

eyes and balance organs; predation with tooth, claw, and sting rapidly became the way of the world. Insertional pain and recoil have a long evolutionary co-history; needles and moxibustion plug straight into this core survival reflex.

Interestingly, you are not born with a coherent recoil reflex. Rather, it takes years for the reflex to mature as the central nervous system (CNS) learns to map and control the moving body. A baby moves when hurt but that movement is poorly coordinated. Maria Fitzgerald of University College London has studied the neurology of recoil in the human baby (Fitzgerald 1998). The baby's nociceptive (pain) fields are larger and smeared in body image, somewhat like the distortion mirrors found at amusement parks. Fine discrimination of hurt is lacking because of the incomplete body mapping by the young brain. Nociceptive fields are significantly more excitable in babies so minor insults can trigger massive reactions. With young children, it is often hard to gauge the severity of an injury as each accident, major and minor, is given a loud and fulsome reaction. Importantly, a noxious insult leaves a long-lasting deleterious neurological impression as the inhibitory pain neurons mature later in development. Pain is easier to inflict and is not filtered or inhibited, as experienced by an adult. Hence the earliest hurts are often the deepest. Babies and young children have yet to develop the accurate neuronal body maps (of which there are many) in the brain that are needed for volitional movement or nuanced recoil (Blakeslee & Blakeslee 2007).

Surprisingly (I thought at first), the Chinese suggest that babies do not have meridians (at this age they suggest the visceral organs dominate); they emerge fully at about 6 years of age. I used to wonder why babies did not have meridians, as every organ, muscle, and bone is anatomically present at birth. Here, I think, the Chinese have left a valuable clue to their mapping of meridians. I hypothesize that meridians emerge from a maturing series of maps of the body schema and recoil reflex. When a child can roll, run, jump, and throw, the brain has mapped the moving body. To construct any map, one of the first priorities is to delineate the various borders involved, a process that I was alert to via the mapping of the CFs.

There is an underlying pattern to recoil once it has matured as a reflex, and the Chinese mapped aspects of this pattern. Meridians are hypothesized to be *'emergent lines of shape control.'* This deceptively important short phrase will take some explanation. My aim here is to offer an explanatory model that addresses three major questions asked of the meridial map. These questions are:

- *Firstly,* meridians are obviously a map of something – what was mapped?
- *Secondly,* the Chinese have located the majority of commonly used acupoints on the meridians – how might they have discovered these seemingly arbitrary points that they attach so much significance to?
- *Thirdly,* why did the Chinese map these enigmatic lines? There are 12 + 2 meridians. Why this number in particular? The meridians are precisely placed on the body. Why do the meridians trace lines that are often complex? A meridian may stop, change direction, and restart. Another meridian may go to one side of a finger or toenail, but not the other. Information is encoded here but what does it tell us and how was it used in medical practice?

The manipulation of body shape is at the heart of this text. The Chinese culture, using thought processes and insights we can only guess at, pondered aspects of shape and form that I also ponder. I have come to respect the meridial map. As I came to terms with what I now think is embedded in the Chinese map I found it informed the nascent CF model. For example, the notion of embedding a sense organ in a CF probably would not have occurred to me without the explicit nudging implied by the meridial map. Western anatomy is an extraordinary undertaking; it is a profound mapping of the body, but its total reliance on material substrates does tend to place conceptual blinkers on one.

A cross-cultural perspective is often of great value in many human endeavors. If a drug company is conducting field research in the Amazonian rainforest to look for a new plant compound to treat disease, the scale of the quest is daunting. In an acre of rainforest there will be thousands of species to assay: leaves, bark, flowers, roots, high canopy, low canopy, and so on – where does one start? Ethnobotany, local botanical knowledge gathered over thousands of years of close association with the living fabric of the rainforest, is the obvious place to start (Cox & Balik 1994). That botanical knowledge is blended with metaphysics, mysticism, magic, and myth. Likewise, it is to be expected that the Chinese map of meridians embeds a particular knowledge that is also surrounded by a context of metaphysics, mysticism, magic, and myth, as was all pre-scientific enquiry into the natural world. The old dark heart is there but so too will there be commonalities that cross the millennia and the cultures as pain and suffering are common to all mankind.

The three questions posited above are big questions that will only ever be partially responded to. The genesis and subsequent refinement of the meridial map has involved many local medical cultures across China, and across millennia, so there is no one interpretation of the meridial map (Scorzon 2003). The decoding of the meridial map proposed here is predicated on insights derived from the CF model and the importance of the archetypal postures. I will assume some familiarity with the Chinese meridial map, as I do not want to rehash the same material found in every text on the meridians of TCM. Many institutions in the Western world now offer university degrees in acupuncture so a theory that links a traditional medical practice to modern norms of biological enquiry and understanding is of obvious value.

If you are not an acupuncturist I still recommend this material to you as it will supplement the preceding chapters. Although I do not dwell on manual technique in this text (as I for one find learning manual technique from a book as plainly difficult as it is to learn tennis strokes from a book), it has become apparent to me that the Chinese used a manual methodology to map meridians and acupoints. That methodology, in part described below, is still applicable today.

THE QUEEN

In Figure 12.2 (redrawn from a photo), the queen termite has helpers that appear to be taking a grip of her swollen anteriolateral body-wall, both left and right of the midline. By pulling together, they must be helping with some physiological function or stabilization. My point here concerns the nature of the line of skin the termite helpers are pulling on. It is a line that is emergent from a myriad of underlying physiological processes that summatively produce the queen's body shape. For example, if the queen loses weight the helpers will need to change their line of grip to get the same pulling effect on her body-wall. It is not a line that is discernable in a cadaver. It is not marked by nerve, blood, muscle, or fascia. It is emergent from a whole, living, pumped-up queen. It is a line that the termite helpers 'feel' for. Meridians have a similar, emergent, 'feel for' quality.

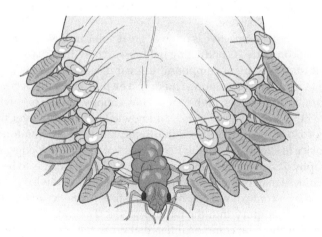

FIG 12.2 A queen termite is facing us with attendants gripping her body-wall, presumably to help with some physiological function. The line they pull on is emergent from the living physiology of the queen. It is a line similar to a meridian.

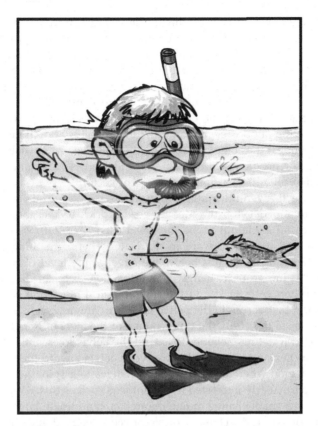

FIG 12.3 The cartoon depicts a person, upright in water with a snorkel, pricked at Ren-12, and shown flexing the body-wall and moving backward away from the penetrating hurt. *Original drawing by MONSTAcartoons (Mark O'Brien), © Elsevier.*

A THOUGHT EXPERIMENT

I will address the reader directly as recoil can be easily imagined. You are standing upright and naked in a deep swimming pool. Your feet are weighted to the pool floor, your head is under the water but a snorkel dispels any panic. In this bizarre situation an experimenter is able to prick any part of your body, without warning, with the tip of something sharp (I have used a fossilized shark tooth). The water acts as a dampening mechanism that steadies and clarifies what happens.

On the body-wall pricking your ventral midline will generally produce flexion and recoil. Moving away from penetrative insult has obvious survival value. To do the opposite, that is to extend your body and move toward the penetrating needle, would be akin to a death wish. Pricking the side of your body will produce a side-bending that is ipsilateral or contralateral. By this I mean a prick to the lateral waist region will make your upper body bend toward the hurt (ipsilateral), whilst a prick to the armpit region of the lateral body-wall will make you bend away from the hurt (contralateral). As an adult, there is no need to think about which direction would be most effective to get away from the needle. A prick from any direction will elicit a movement that will try to minimize the penetrative exposure to hurt.

A needle to the midline of your low back will extend you and move you forward so that you move away from the pain. The CF model helps understand the mass recruitment of muscles that the recoil will elicit. In this case the whole dorsal domain of the dorso/ventro contractile field (D/V-CF) would contract to extend the body, from the eyes elevating to para-spinal extension, to the pubococcygeus, and the lower rectus abdominis extending the caudal body. Lines emerge on the body-wall that, when stabbed with a sharp tooth or needled with a 2000-year-old Chinese acupuncture needle (read blunt), will initiate a similar movement vector.

Let us use the ventral midline meridian – the Ren Mai meridian – to demonstrate and develop the idea. A needle prick to the abdominal wall below the costal angle but above the navel (Ren-12/11/10/9) would cause you to flex and move backward in the water. Then something interesting happens. Needling Ren-6 just below the navel at the level of a belt buckle marks the beginning of a change in the direction of recoil. Because of the lumbar curve in your back, and the embryological migration of the caudal muscles from the sacrum to the pelvic floor, you are now as likely to extend your pelvis as to flex it. By the time you are at the level of Ren-4 (below the belt buckle) it is definitely better to extend the pelvis to escape the penetrating insult, as flexion at Ren-4 will move your pelvis toward the needle. Here we have a region where a spinal flexion changes to a spinal extension. Scientists are particularly interested in phenomena such as this, a form of phase transition, as a small change in one parameter can initiate large changes in the system under study. Here, a couple of centimeters change the direction of a whole-organism movement pattern from flexion to extension. Understanding these critical tipping points of a system gives one more control over the system.

The Chinese gave great importance to areas of the body where movement fields change character. Spleen-21 (phi chih ta lo or Dabao), an acupoint that was historically important (Lu & Needham 1980), is another of these movement field inversion loci on the body-wall. The acupoint is found on the lateral body-wall, the mid-axillary line, sixth or seventh intercostal space. A noxious stimulus below Spleen-21 will initiate ipsilateral side-bending whereas a noxious stimulus above Spleen-21 will initiate contralateral side-bending. So Spleen-21 was probably recognized as important because it represents a border region on the lateral body-wall between dorsal and ventral, and left/right side-bending. One of its clinical indications is whole-body pain. I imagine a moxa cone that was allowed to burn the skin on this sensitive area of the body would really hurt; that hurt would affect a nodal region of one or more of the brain's maps of the body. Pain is a CNS phenomenon so a burn here would spread its nociceptive effect over a wide area of your brain's internal mapping of the body, and reduce the perception of other pains for some time. If the patient was suffering from intractable severe pain this moxibustion treatment might have offered a form of respite. I suspect the acupoint may have fallen out of favour because too many cases of what we now call a pneumothorax occurred because of acupuncture needles deflating a lung.

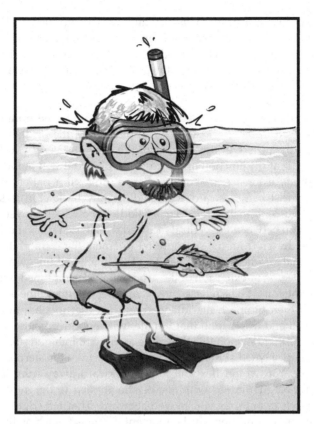

FIG 12.4 A thought experiment comically depicts extension of the pelvis when Ren-4 is pricked. *Original drawing by MONSTAcartoons (Mark O'Brien). © Elsevier.*

With knowledge of CFs it becomes possible to comprehend the biomechanics involved in recoil. A sharp (tooth) stab to the dorsal body that spans from left rib angle to right rib angle will initiate extension, with slight variations on the theme depending on the point of contact. Likewise, the ventral domain of the dorso/ventro contractile field (D/V-CF) is a broad river of contractility that, if pierced, will flex the body. The lateral contractile field (L-CF) will side-bend the body when pricked, with flexion or extension usually thrown into the biomechanical mix as the lateral border is vaguely defined on the soma and in the brain.

Needling the borders between the CFs will challenge the brain's sensory/ movement maps so a mixture of both CFs will fire, which the helical contractile field (H-CF) can help us to understand, as twisting is a biomechanical compound of both lateral flexion and flexion/extension. Thus the intermediate lines between the D/V-CF and the L-CF are seen as initiators of twisting movement. The meridial map suggested the modelling of the limb CFs as emerging from helical biomechanics.

Needling the limbs and face whilst standing in the water will reveal more of the transition zones where a small change in needle location will initiate a big change in movement direction. Limbs are further discussed below so, here, a quick consideration of the face is appropriate. When standing upright and looking ahead, a prick to the lateral jaw will produce a side-bending ipsilaterally, but above the zygomatic arch, contralateral side-bending is the face-saving thing to do. The zygomatic arch of the temporal bone straddles the border between side-bending toward or side-bending away from the needle via the ipsilateral or contralateral sternocleidomastoid (SCM) and the lateral suboccipital muscles.

The face is a highly innervated region so a needle to the front of the face will be nuanced in its effect. A needle applied from the bridge of the nose to the tip of the nose will flex the top of the neck and send you backward, whilst a needle at the junction of the nose and philtrum will initiate a powerful whole-body extension movement. For example, if a patient presents to an acupuncturist bent forward with midline low back pain this acupoint (Renzhong Du-26, translated as Man's Middle) is often employed.

The junction between the ventral face and the lateral face is marked by the straight line drawn from the supraorbital foramen, the infraorbital foramen, and the mental foramen of the lower jaw. This junctional line, when needled, will initiate flexion or extension of the head and neck, combined with rotation away from the hurt. The Chinese considered this emergent line and incorporated it into their Stomach meridian, a meridian that touches many loci on the body-wall and lower limb that initiate twisting movements (the H-CF).

We shall further develop this thought experiment. Imagine standing in the pool and being needled at Ren-12 (about half-way from the sternocostal angle to the navel). You would flex and move backward away from the danger. What cannot be guaranteed with one needle applied to the midline is your drift to the left or right as you move backward. That left/right drift arises from small initial conditions at the moment of impact, such as the direction of your gaze or one leg more weighted than the other. How might that left/right drift be controlled? To be able to predict flex and send you *straight* backward the experimenter would need to use two needles. Two needles, one on either side of Ren-12 (i.e. Kidney-19, a point that is about half the width of your thumb lateral to the ventral midline), would still flex the body and make it move away in the water, but now with added directional control. Using pressure that is more penetrative on the left or right needle, recoil away can be left/right influenced. In effect, this is a form of 'border control.'

BORDER CONTROL

Borders are important in all arenas of life, from the microscopic to the macroscopic. A border needs two semi-independent zones or membranes in order to effectively control movement across domains. For example, every animal cell is surrounded by a lipid bilayer that is formed by two sheets of phospholipid molecules arranged back-to-back. Lipids are free to move in the plane of their own layer, making the structure a liquid crystal that is both flexible but structurally robust, as it is neither a solid nor a liquid (Kingsland 2000). Extracellular material has to negotiate two walls of lipid in order to reach the intracellular domain. A non-biological example of border control is that of a kite. A single string allows one to control height. Two strings allow far more control of the kite's flight as a border is controlled. Likewise one hand on the top of a car's steering wheel will offer poor control of the vehicle as the hand will tend to constantly fall to the left or right. Two hands that span the midline border of the steering wheel will offer a much safer grip of the wheel with more directional control. Earlier walls (which date to about 208 BC) preceded the Great Wall of China, so the Chinese were very border conscious at a critical stage in the mapping of something we now call meridians. The concept of border control is essential to the decoding hypothesis presented.

THE LEECH

John Lewis and William Kristan (Kristan & Lewis 1998a,b; see also Howlett 1998 for a summary of the research), using a leech as a model organism, have studied the neurophysiology of recoil. This work is essential to a modern understanding of the meridial map. The leech was chosen as a model organism as it has relatively few sensory neurons distributed around the body-wall. The sensory neurons are patterned so that there are four overlapping sensory fields that cover the circumference of the leech body. A pinprick that elicits recoil will usually fire two sensory neurons because of the generous overlapping of sensory territory. These two sensory neurons feed down to interneurons that summate the neuronal data input, and inform the motor neurons to move the appropriate part of the body-wall away via specific muscle contraction. What Lewis and Kristan discovered was the mathematical ability of the interneuronal layer. These nerve cells can, in effect, add, subtract, compute sines and cosines, and manipulate trigonometric identities that would challenge a 15-year-old with a calculator. Apparently a leech interneuron knows $\cos(\varphi - \theta)$. Lewis and Kristan suspect all higher organisms use overlapping sensory fields and an almost hard-wired sense of trigonometry to avoid penetrative insult.

With four overlapping sensory fields, the leech would conceptually need eight longitudinal lines to control its four borders. With eight emergent lines of control, the leech could be predictably manipulated using pinpricks.

SHAPE CONTROL – PART I

How many emergent lines of shape control are needed to predictably control subtle human shape, our functional morphology? Borders will need to be identified and then controlled using lines (meridians) on either side of that border. The CF model identifies primary mammalian movement fields as flexion/extension, side-bending, twisting left or right, squeezing/sucking, and limb fields. Each field borders other fields and the fields are profoundly interactive. To control subtle human body shape – predictably – emergent lines of shape control would need to be placed as follows:

- The dorsal and ventral midline. Vertebrates are bilaterally symmetrical – the midline representation is mandatory (Ren Mai and Du Mai meridians).
- To border control the dorsal and ventral midline, bilateral/paraxial lines would need to be erected (inner Bladder meridian and the Kidney meridian).

163

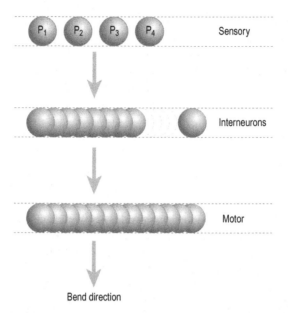

FIG 12.5 Four overlapping sensory fields covering the circumference of the leech feed neuronal data to the interneurons. The interneurons are the mathematical geniuses. *Adapted from Howlett 1998.*

- The lateral body-wall has an indistinct dorsal/ventral border. To control laterality, criss-crossed lines need to be placed near the dorsal and ventral margins of the L-CF (Gall Bladder and Liver meridians).
- The Chinese control the radial contractile field (R-CF) via the Girdling (also known as the Dai Mai) meridian. This is the only horizontal meridian. From a manipulation of shape perspective it is essential. It is traditionally placed as a loose belt around the waist because squeezing the body-wall above would compromise breathing, whilst below the waist, the ilia and the robust sacroiliac joints do not allow a radial compression.
- Helical movements are introduced when you needle four intermediate lines on the body-wall, as helical biomechanics are a compound of flexion/extension and left/right side-bending. These four intermediate lines are marked by the rib angles on the thorax and the lateral raphe of the thoracolumbar region of the dorsal body. On the ventral body-wall the intermediate line is marked on the face by the line linking the supraorbital, the infraorbital, and the mental foramen, the costochondral junction and the linea semilunaris of the abdominal wall (lateral Bladder meridian and the Spleen/Stomach meridians). Note that erecting lines of border control on either side of the intermediate body-wall is unnecessary as the twisting movements they are capable of initiating are derived from the D/V-CF and the L-CF. Extra lines placed on either side of the intermediate lines would offer no additional control of movement.
- Limbs derive from fins. Fins are optimally placed on the body-wall of a fish to control pitch, yaw, and roll. Small movements of a fin create large changes in direction. Terrestrial vertebrate limbs became stout and

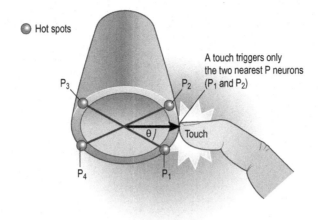

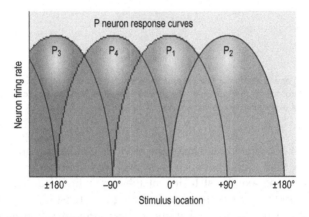

FIG 12.6 Usually a touch will fire two P neurons Each P neuron will send neuronal data to the interneurons. The leech has four borders between the sensory domains, therefore eight emergent meridians are needed for shape control of a leech. *Adapted from Howlett 1998.*

propulsive but in essence still control movement. The embryonic limb bud is paddle shaped and is described as having a pre-axial border (thumb side), a post-axial border (little finger side), and ventral/dorsal axial lines that mark the midline of the limb bud. Six lines are needed to control the limb bud shape. Two lines are needed to control the leading edge (the pre-axial border) of the limb bud (Lung and Large Intestine/ Spleen and Stomach). Two lines are needed to control the trailing edge (the post-axial border) of the limb bud (Heart and Small Intestine/ Kidney and Bladder). Two lines are also needed to mark the ventral/ dorsal midline of the limb bud (Pericardium and Sanjiao/Liver and Gall Bladder). These six lines allow accurate shape control of the embryonic limb bud.

Note how embryology describes a border, and the Chinese place two lines on either side of that border, and acknowledge this in their theoretical model (see Fig. 2.15). Looking at the adult limb this pattern is far less obvious, especially in the leg. The Chinese must have pondered long and

165

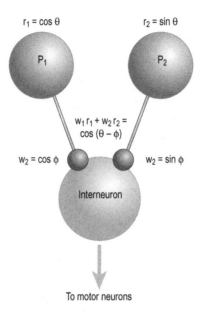

$r_1 = \cos \theta$

$r_2 = \sin \theta$

P₁

P₂

$w_1 r_1 + w_2 r_2 = \cos (\theta - \phi)$

$w_2 = \cos \phi$

$w_2 = \sin \phi$

Interneuron

To motor neurons

FIG 12.7 P₁ and P₂ send information regarding the velocity and strength of the insult to the interneuron that computes the optimum signal to feed forward to the motor neuron. As every interneuron knows, $\cos (\phi - \theta)$. *Adapted from Howlett 1998.*

hard about how they could map the obvious similarities and the profound differences they found between arms and legs. Embryologically, the lower limb has a long axis twist to it that the upper limb bud does not experience. Due to the internal rotation and long axis twist of the lower limb the quadriceps of the leg is analogous to the triceps of the arm. Thus, dorsal moiety muscle migrates to the ventral aspect of the leg. Note how the Chinese have placed the Stomach meridian, a Yang (dorsal body) meridian, on the ventral surface of the leg and torso. I suggest the crossing of the leg Yin meridians at Spleen-6, the crossing of the Bladder meridian behind the knee, and the crossing of the Stomach meridian at the hip joint, all suggest this attempt to map the long axis rotation of the leg. The arm meridians, in contrast, are parallel so they do not cross, reflecting the less complexly rotated embryological development.

Although the limb borders become obscured later in development they are nevertheless important to structure and function. When people walk and run, look for arms or legs that seem to be too internally or externally rotated. The Chinese call the acupoints on either side of the patella tendon the 'eyes of the knees,' possibly because the eyes should be focused and look ahead. Normal limb biomechanics allow the borders to assume their correct placement in the movements of life. Skilful manual therapy, corrective exercises and acupuncture all help tune bodies to norms that are biomechanically efficient and economical.

The model thus predicts the dorsal and ventral midline as two lines, four para-axial lines to control the dorsal/ventral midlines, four widely spaced lines to control the indistinct lateral body-wall, and four lines that are intermediately placed to initiate helical movement. Therefore, is it surprising the

Chinese describe their meridian system as having 2 midline meridians and a further 12 principal meridians?

However, if you count around the torso, the Chinese actually map 16 meridians, as the Bladder meridian was divided into 2 meridians but named as only 1. What might this mean? The Chinese medical theorists recognized the importance of the nipple line, and the need for its representation. Breasts and suckling lips are unique mammalian attributes that are essential to childhood survival – without a wet-nurse you starve. Embryologically, the nipple line, in its early embryonic period as part of the Wolffian ridge, is intermediate in its placement on the body-wall near the Spleen meridian. During subsequent development, the arms rotate in a lateral direction and the legs rotate in an internal direction, pulling the skin and the nipple line medially (see Fig. 2.10). The now displaced nipple line needed to be represented (Stomach meridian). Hence 16 meridians pass down the torso.

The correspondence between traditional Chinese meridial theory and the decoding hypothesis is substantial. The decoding hypothesis presented here makes sense of much of the arcane information packaged with meridians. Three examples follow.

THE INTERIOR–EXTERIOR RELATIONSHIP

Pairs of meridians are traditionally coupled together in what is called an 'exterior–interior' relationship. Each limb has six meridians so three pairs are described, the pairs linking a Yang and a Yin meridian of the anterior, middle, and posterior portions of the limbs. In other words, the meridians are coupled across the pre-axial and post-axial borders and the midlines of the limbs. They are coupled together across borders because both are needed to control the border. One without the other is like a car able to turn only to the left. When I studied acupuncture theory the internal–external relationship was presented as yet another arcane fact. Appreciating how coupled meridians act to control a border gives the relationship new meaning. One can then ask how the Chinese used border control on the limbs in the clinical situation.

THE SIX-CHANNEL PAIRING

This pairing of meridian couples (for example) a Yang meridian of the anterior arm to a Yang meridian of the anterior leg. Using embryological language it is obvious that the Chinese have coupled a dorsal (Yang) pre-axial border on the arm (thumb side) being analogous to a dorsal (Yang) pre-axial border of the leg (big toe side). The Chinese have matched lines on the arm and leg for what I suggest to be the pre-axial border, the post-axial border, and dorsal/ventral limb midline. Because of this important pairing the Chinese considered how they would link the arm meridians to the leg meridians. Analysis of the meridial map from this perspective yields some interesting associations. The six-channel pairing required a deep analysis of the movement patterns found between the arms and legs, via the torso. Two thousand years later biomechanical models of human movement, robotics, and computer animation are asking similar questions.

The Lung and Large Intestine, and Spleen and Stomach meridians are paired meridians that control the pre-axial border of the limbs. From a CF perspective these meridians appear to then map helical biodynamics on the torso. The meridians seem to suggest that the limbs' pre-axial border exert a torque effect on the torso as the meridians track intermediate lines on the torso, lines that if needled will tend to induce twisting movements. A fish will use the four-fin pre-axial borders as leading-edge foils in a fluid medium to direct movement. How one attempts to understand this relationship between pectoral and pelvic fins via the CF model is a question I would not have considered if not for the Chinese meridial theory that already attempts to answer this question. Possibly the martial arts helped inform their model. In the martial arts, wristlocks are a powerful way of controlling movement. They are applied unilaterally, usually to the medial or lateral hand, and will take the opponent down to the floor in swooping, twisting movements. Meridians map considerable thought and reflection on the nature of human movement.

The Heart and Small Intestine, and Kidney and Bladder meridians are paired meridians that control the post-axial border of the limbs. They appear to then map the dorsal/ventral region of the torso (with a hint of connection to helical dynamics). Meridial theory thus links the trailing edge of the limbs to the para-midline of the torso. Again, the martial arts come to mind, as a karate strike from the ulnar border of the hand is very powerful, unlike a strike with the thumb side of the limb that would just break the striker's wrist. The force generated by the ulnar hand strike is transmitted and dissipated in the striker's body via the middle of the torso.

The Pericardium and Sanjiao, and Liver and Gall Bladder meridians are paired meridians that track the midlines of the limbs. Here, the pattern of relationship is more complex. The Pericardium and Sanjiao of the arm link to the midline of the torso, as expected from this understanding: midline of upper limb to midline of torso. However, the Liver and Gall Bladder of the lower limb midline link to the lateral body-wall. I suspect this relationship is derived from the postures used to palpate these midline leg meridians, as described later in the text.

I am reminded of my math homework at high school. The guts of a math problem are considerably easier to work out when one has the answer at the back of the text. As the Chinese meridial map continues lines from the leading and trailing edge of the limbs back to the torso, in a non-random way, it is interesting to consider their finding as they are a historical record of a prolonged, insightful thought process about the nature of movement. These early attempts at understanding their thought process are necessarily speculative.

DEEP MERIDIANS – THE INTERIOR PATHWAYS

Deep meridians connect the superficial 12 + 2 meridians to the interior of the body. Deep meridians are fascinating and conceptually comprehensible from the perspective of the manipulation of shape. The Chinese give real importance to these deep pathways because they are often used to explain why an acupoint on a superficial meridian will affect a remote area of the body or the viscera. For example, Pericardium-6 on the forearm is used to treat nausea and vomiting because (it is said) the Pericardium deep meridian originates in the middle of the chest where it will continue via the midline to the lower abdomen. Hence Pericardium-6 treats nausea and vomiting that originates in the middle of the torso.

Meridians are depicted as being bilaterally symmetrical. Each meridian has a distinct left and a distinct right – only at the mouth and anal/genitals are the 12 meridians routinely depicted as being crossed. CF modelling leads one to consider where muscles decuss as they form the warp and weft of the body's musculature. Meridians via the deep channels are also comprehensively networked across the midline, particularly the ventral midline. When the Stomach channel sends a deep channel to the ventral midline at Ren-12 and 13 it means this meridian meets its contralateral counterpart and thus the meridian can be drawn as decussing. Many other meridians send deep branches to the midline where they can meet and therefore cross. If the meridial map was drawn in this way it would look quite different, far more complex, but surprisingly similar to a new anatomical map of the abdominal wall.

The 38th edition of *Gray's Anatomy* (Williams 1995) devotes 11 pages to the abdominal wall musculature. At the end of this classic description it is noted that a newer, highly detailed map of the musculature is available. Nabil Rizk described the musculature of the abdominal wall in unprecedented detail (Rizk 1980). He had 114 fresh abdominal walls delivered to his lab, 76 from men and women, the remainder from African mammals. Over hundreds of hours, he meticulously tracked individual muscle fibers. Buried in his 13-page article is a schema of the abdominal wall, a couple of diagrams that in effect summarize the PhD he earned with this work. Rizk identifies seven vertical lines where the trilaminar body-wall muscles cross paths and form the fascial sheath of the rectus abdominis. Two thousand years ago the Chinese ran seven lines down the abdominal wall in exactly the same layout (the midline, two para-midlines, two lines on the middle of the rectus abdominis, and two lines to mark the lateral border of the rectus abdominis). If you needed to control biodynamics across the abdominal wall, knowledge of these lines is mandatory. An analogy here would be a hypothetical need to control traffic coming into Wellington, New Zealand. Two motorways converge to enter the city, which terminate at the airport, whilst all sea traffic needs to enter via the heads of the harbour. Control these three choke points and 99% of all traffic into Wellington is accounted for. Meridians are emergent lines that control movement and, like the CFs, are comprehensively interconnected and decussed across the midline.

Viewing meridians as being only bilateral and symmetrical is a disservice to the considerable thought and clinical insight that was embedded in the map. Using acupoints on the right to treat left-sided pain is well accepted in TCM, and the meridial map details how those patterns of relationship may be tracked.

Deep meridians also link the superficial meridians to the visceral organs and the brain. The Chinese saw clinical relationships between patterns of presenting clinical symptoms and palpable trigger points that linked the palpable outside body to the deep body. These relationships came to be formalized later in the historical development of the meridial map, with each meridian being named after a widely defined viscera. Linking a line on the surface of the body to a specific visceral organ probably reflects an attempt to conceptually unify the acu-moxa and manual therapy practices with herbal medicine theory.

Bioscience has recognized viscero-somatic reflexes and other patterns of referred pain, but the relationship is usually a non-linear one. Pain of a visceral origin converges on interneurons in the spinal cord but those same interneurons also receive input from the musculoskeletal system. But as I have discovered with the CF model, it is tempting to push a model too far. The Chinese may well have done this with the meridial map. For example, the Large Intestine meridian is not used to treat the large intestine, and the Triple Heater meridian needed a fictitious visceral organ to be created as all the palpable visceral organs had been allotted to meridians.

THE LICHENIFORM RASH

At this stage I will introduce an article that originally appeared in the *European Journal of Oriental Medicine* (James 1993). Dr Richard James described a case of a 25-year-old woman who presented to the dermatology clinic of a London teaching hospital. She had a rash that had been present for 1 month, was distributed in one line on the arm and one line on the leg, and each line was about 0.5–1.0 cm width. The lines consisted of red, flat-topped papules a few millimeters across, and were licheniform and itchy. They were accurately drawn and discussed by the staff at the clinic, as they did not seem to conform to dermatomes. An acupuncturist would immediately have seen a close similarity with the Kidney and the Pericardium meridians.

Dr James then undertook a literature review to see if other cases of the meridian-like rashes had been documented. One researcher (Blaschko 1901) had carefully drawn about 200 rashes of all kinds, some of which Dr James saw as being similar to the case he described. In summary Dr James suggests the concept of meridians may not be redundant as they might be the best working hypothesis to explain a number of phenomena, including those strange skin rashes.

As the brain maps the body during normal childhood development, one of the first requirements is to delineate fields of movement and the borders between movement patterns. Deep in the brain there are many maps of the body, maps that are interrelated and networked together to form a cohesive sense of self. One of those maps is referenced (I hypothesize) to the pre- and post-axial borders, and the ventral axial lines of the limb buds. Very occasionally a neuro-irritant must upset neurons that collaborate to form the map, hence the reflex manifestation of a meridian-like skin rash that does not follow the more usual dermatomal pattern.

HAND-HOLDS – THE ORIGIN OF MANY ACUPOINTS

To effectively move a patient's body, manual hand-holds are employed. A hand-hold is a specific placing of the practicioner's hands on the patient's body to facilitate or support movement in a specific direction. Manual

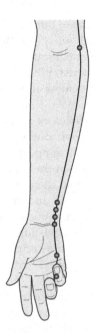

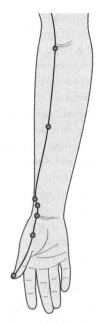

FIG 12.8 **Heart meridian** Note the acupoint at the anteriomedial elbow followed by no acupoint until four acupoints are depicted just proximal to the medial wrist.

FIG 12.9 **Lung meridian** Note the acupoint (Lung-6) that is just proximal to the half-way point between the ventro-lateral elbow and the lateral wrist. How did the Chinese discern this acupoint?

technique teaches one to palpate (to examine the body via a sense of touch), and to use hand-holds to manipulate soft tissues and joints. TCM teaches one to identify specific loci on the body that have been identified as being particularly important to the practice of acupuncture. A combination of these manual skills has proved to be useful to help understand the manual methodology used by the Chinese when they mapped the enigmatic meridians and acupoints.

I will describe this manual methodology using two meridians on the arm as they demonstrate the principle which can then be extended to all the meridians. The Heart meridian tracks down the medial ventral arm or, from an embryological perspective, the ventral aspect of the post-axial border. The Lung meridian tracks down the lateral ventral arm, the ventral aspect of the pre-axial border of the limb bud. The contrast between the acupoints on these two meridians from the elbow distally is the subject discussed here.

The Heart meridian has one acupoint on the medial end of the transverse cubital crease of medial ventral elbow (Heart-3). Then the meridian courses distally down the forearm to the medial aspect of the wrist, where four acupoints are closely spaced just proximal to the wrist (Heart-4/5/6/7). There are no acupoints between the elbow and these four acupoints near the wrist.

171

The Lung meridian, in contrast, has a similar course but from the ventral lateral elbow (Lung-5), then distal to the lateral wrist via the forearm. However, the Lung meridian has an acupoint, Lung-6, located just proximal to the midpoint between the elbow and the lateral wrist. Why does the Heart meridian have no intervening acupoints between the elbow and wrist whereas the Lung meridian does with Lung-6?

I often mused upon such questions. The hand-holds of manual therapy answer many of these questions. A hand-hold in this context refers to the manual application of force to predictably move or support the patient's body in a specific direction. Hand-holds are the stock-in-trade of the manual therapies and the martial arts. An experienced manual therapy practicioner or martial artist spends years learning, both consciously and unconsciously, the art of taking grips on another person to direct motion. Those grips can change the shape of the recipient overtly as in twisting the torso or limbs, or the grips may exert very subtle effects on the recipient, such as used in cranial techniques where intention is imparted with very light pressures.

The Heart meridian, taken as a whole, represents hand-holds to internally rotate or pronate the arm. Heart-3 is a strong manual promotor of internal rotation of the arm as the medial epicondyle of the elbow has sensitive soft tissues and neurovascular bundles that hurt when compressed against the bone. The Heart meridian then offers no hand-holds until the practitioner reaches the medial wrist where one is able to use three fingers to grip the distal/ventral ulnar bone to pronate the arm. Two thousand plus years ago a Chinese acupuncturist/manual therapist gripped these distal medial wrist points on the Heart meridian with three fingers and noted four acupoints around the grip offered by the three fingers. Here we have a strong hand-hold that will pronate the arm whereas, proximal to this region, the ulna is able to roll easily toward supination as the hand-holds are not grip-effective on the underlying bone.

The Lung meridian, when manually manipulated (in contrast to the Heart meridian), externally rotates or supinates the arm. Lung-5 is a powerful hand-hold for external rotation as, again, sensitive neuromuscular bundles are compressed against the bone – it is very painful to resist. Then, as one palpates the Lung meridian distal to the elbow, the hand-holds are ineffec- tive until one reaches Lung-6 where the radius becomes a firm, often tender hand-hold to push against if the patient tries to turn the arm internally against the hand-hold. It is easy to convincingly demonstrate this effect in contrast to the many words needed to describe it. The Lung meridian is a series of hand-holds that form an emergent line of palpation for external rotation of the arm, with Lung-6 discerned because it offers a particularily effective locus for a digital pressure against the ventral radius, as do the Lung acupoints at the wrist.

The same principle can be used to show why the Chinese track meridians to one side or the other of the finger- and toenails. Information of a type is encoded here. Nail points are extremely tender if needled or pushed with the practitioner's fingernail; in fact, a needle to these points has a pain of fire-like intensity. Heart-9 is located on the radial side of the little fingernail.

Placing Heart-9 on the radial side of the little finger nail bed means it is a strong promotor of pronation, as is the rest of the meridian. If the meridian had been tracked to the ulnar side of the little finger nail bed, as at first glance would look look more likely, it would promote supination of the hand and arm.

Lung-11 illustrates a thought process at work two millenia ago. The Lung meridian tracks to the radial side of the thumb's nail, hence medially rotating the thumb if needled. All the rest of the meridian externally rotates the upper limb so we have a mismatch not found in the other meridial nail points. I suspect the Chinese noted the unique nature of the thumb's carpometacarpal joint, a saddle-shaped joint that allows 3 degrees of rotation. This unique joint (acting with the metacarpo-phalangeal joint) allows the thumb to flex and extend, abduct and adduct, and an axial rotation (also called pronation) that facilitates opposition of the thumb to the other fingers. Opposition allows the thumb pad to touch any other finger pad so that the grips we use in daily life are enabled. Orthopedic practice has learnt that the hand must not be cast in an open posture as the functional pronation of the thumb is so important. The pronation of the thumb is essential to normal hand function and I suggest the deliberate placing of Lung-11 on the radial nail bed reflects this functional priority. So the arm can be externally rotated but the thumb must be able to oppose the other fingers if the hand/arm is to be functional.

Thousands of years of manual therapy and the cultivation of martial arts facilitated a profound mapping of hand-holds. As discussed in limb development, small changes in limb internal/external rotation can cause large changes in bodily movement because the fingers and toes are so densely represented on the cortex. A fish changes pitch via small changes to the angles of the fins; so too, I suspect that small changes in the limb's ability to internally/externally rotate reflect deeper physiological biases. Early Chinese doctors, with no recourse to imaging techniques, took a case history and then palpated the body. Over millenia they discerned patterns, often derived from a manual intimacy with the body, that they then condensed into their meridial map.

SHAPE CONTROL – PART 2

Meridians are emergent from a whole living organism that is able to react coherently to a noxious stimulus. When an organism is too tired (Qi deficient) the meridians will diminish. No energy – no recoil. At death, meridians depart, so they will not be found in a cadaver. They are not a distinct biological tissue and this is why they have proved to be so elusive to bioscience. Meridians, it is hypothesized, allow subtle shape to be predictably manipulated.

The key word is 'predictably.' Chinese medical theorists mapped the minimum number of lines, in carefully discerned locations, to offer a high degree of control of subtle shape by using a three-dimensional pattern of pinpricks. Morphology, the shape of biological form, is tremendously important. For example, a small deformation of heart valve shape can have profound long-term effects on cardiovascular health. Eddies and crosscurrents are created in the hemodynamic that gradually erode the patency of the cardiovascular system. Likewise, a small change in the shape of the eye lens will affect vision. For many years I have ridden motorbikes and I am constantly impressed by the year-on-year power increase from the same cubic centimeter (cc) engine size. Again it is subtle changes in the shape of the combustion area, valve angles, etc., that enhance combustion and gas flow. Particularly in biology it is not just a local change in shape that is important, rather it is the harmonious integration of multiple shapes that is important – that is emergent tune.

Once the Chinese had mapped a way of predictably influencing shape they looked for patterns of shape distortion associated with disease, for example as Western medicine has done with heart valves and the shape of the eye lens. The genius of the Chinese was to then use this map to influence subtle body shape and function. From this perspective, acupoint combinations to treat clinical syndromes are a form of three-dimensional shape manipulation. Shape and physiological function are closely coupled. To treat a condition, acupuncturists use a 'point combination' that usually employs 10–20 needles on the head, torso, arms, and legs. Like clouds moving slowly across the sky, point combinations change with disease and during the course of a disease.

We all have a feeling for being 'in shape' or 'out of shape.' It is often subtle. I learnt my TCM point prescriptions via small drawings that depicted in caricature the syndrome I was trying to memorize. The syndrome caricatures had the swollen bellies, the weak knees, the red eyes, etc. that depicted the condition. When point prescriptions are seen in this light they appear to be an exercise in three-dimensional shape normalization.

Lung-Qi deficiency, as an example, is a coalescence of signs and symptoms discerned by the Chinese. Clinical manifestations of this syndrome include shortness of breath, a weak voice, and a bright-white complexion. A classic point combination used to treat Lung-Qi deficiency would include acupoints like Ren-17, Lung-1 and 7, Bladder-13, Ren-6, and Stomach-36.

Ren-17 is the first point needled; it acts as a nodal point about which all subsequent biodynamic movement will pivot. Embryologically, the lungs start as a midline bud off the gut tube; the bud bifurcates and gradually courses around the chest wall to nearly meet at the ventral midline. Lung-1 will tend to take the shoulders backward, as deep to this acupoint lies the brachial plexus. Lung-7 and Lung-9 would externally rotate the upper limb and lift the viscera within the raised chest wall, via and empowered by a long lever effect. If pushed from behind via Du-12 and Bladder-13, the effect on the upper torso is localized and upper spinal extension is enhanced. Ren-6 below the navel establishes another midline nodal point. If the upper body is to expand and be externally rotated (taking the lung fields with it) the lower body must do the opposite as shape can be changed but volume cannot. Stomach-36 (just below the lateral knee) will internally rotate the legs with this summating as a squeezing in the region of Ren-6, thus facilitating the upper body to expand. Repeatedly using this point combination encourages and conditions a change in the body's functional shape. Combined with dietary advice, herbs, and exercises, this treatment may well have pulled the patient back from the brink that in our modern world could lead to antibiotics, inhalers, steroids, and nebulizers.

MOVEMENT, LIMB BUDS, AND MERIDIANS

Table 12.1 shows a schema that links the CFs to the meridians of TCM. Hundreds of years of collective clinical experience, derived from methodologies available at the time, coalesced to form the meridial map. Unlike the impression given by the title of Ted Kaptchuck's book *Chinese Medicine; The Web that Has No Weaver* (Kaptchuck 1983) that implies the meridians are just a given, I see considerable human thought embedded in this old map.

The meridial map is like a complex text that has been extensively modified by many contributors over a long time period. It will not easily give up its secrets, and at best we can only approximate the original rhyme and reason that generated the map as we know it today.

Six meridians will be briefly discussed as a way of trying to understand what the meridial map may be trying to convey to us in this new millennium. To help with this, there are photographs of postures that may have facilitated the hand-holds used to discern the meridians and acupoints as meridians make little sense when referenced only to the 'anatomical posture.' Each posture exposes different information about the structure and function of the body. Loss of ease in these primary postures can indicate patterns of distress or sub-optimal function. The archetypal postures that have been introduced as a way of assessing biomechanical tune have helped guide this enquiry. When one loses access to these postures, trigger points (TPs) often emerge at the site of the hand-hold that would move the body toward the restricted direction. TPs become predictable to palpation. Their manifestation has rhyme and reason – they do not just appear. Again this is a type of knowledge that is derived from a manual methodology, just as good tennis play is emergent from years of a particular practice that is hard to scientifically box or reduce to numbers. But like a good tennis stroke, the effect is easy to demonstrate.

Table 12.1 Contractile fields and the meridians of TCM		
Part of body	**Field**	**Meridian**
Torso	Flexion/extension	Conception and Kidney Governing and Bladder
	Side-bending	Gall Bladder and Liver
	Helical	Stomach and Spleen
	Radial	Girdling (or Dai Mai)
Fore limb	Ventral axial line	Pericardium
	Dorsal axial line	Sanjiao
	Pre-axial border	Lung and Large Intestine
	Post-axial border	Heart and Small Intestine
Hind limb	Ventral axial line	Liver
	Dorsal axial line	Gall Bladder
	Pre-axial border	Stomach and Spleen
	Post-axial border	Kidney and Bladder

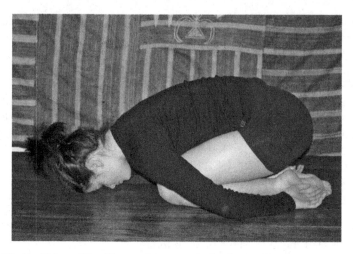

FIG 12.10 Du Mai meridian The meridian is stretched and exposed in this posture.

GOVERNING VESSEL (DU MAI MERIDIAN)

- It maps the dorsal midline.
- It originates in the lower abdomen as a deep meridian. Two thousand years later, embryology tracks the dorsal muscle precursor to the lower abdomen via the pelvic floor.
- It wraps around the external genitalia and the anus to emerge between the anus and the coccyx (as does the streaming mesoderm), to then ascend the spine to the brain and the vertex of the head. From the vertex of the head the meridian sends extensions of itself to the lateral region of the skull and brain, probably because the midline can exist only when supported by a lateral stability. Imagine a ridge tent with no lateral guy ropes: it would not stay up for long. The meridian then continues to track the midline to the nose and philtrum, to terminate at the superior frenulum inside the mouth. Again the embryology is congruent with this mapping as the teeth emerge from the first pharyngeal arch that is, by definition, a ventral body structure, so the Du Mai meridian is congruent with embryonic dorsal tissue. Thus the Chinese accurately mapped the dorsal body from the caudal pole to the cephalic pole.
- The acupoints have been selected as they activate key spinal segments that lift or extend the body.

CONCEPTION VESSEL (REN MAI MERIDIAN)

- It maps the ventral midline.
- It originates in the lower abdomen (and the uterus in females) to emerge superficially at the perineal body, and ascends the ventral midline to the mentolabial groove above the chin. From here, a deep meridian encircles the mouth to meet with the Governing Vessel. The Chinese map is again

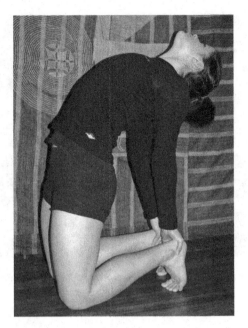

FIG 12.11 **Ren Mai meridian** This is a posture that may have been used to map the meridian.

congruent with the embryology. The mouth is a ventral body structure. The lower incisors have an innervation that crosses the midline so dentists will often need to nerve block both sides of the jaw when working on these teeth.

- Lateral stability of the midline is again addressed by the meridian sending deep aspects of itself to radiate from the ziphoid region over the upper abdomen, and another deep extension meets the eyes. All mammals link the nose and eyes to the genitals.

BLADDER MERIDIAN

- It maps para-axial lines of border control over the dorsal midline of the spine. On the lower limb the meridian maps the post-axial border.
- The Bladder meridian is a long meridian that on the head and torso tracks the dorsal aspect of the D/V-CF. It starts at the inner canthus of the eyes. From a martial arts/manual therapy perspective the inner canthus is a vulnerable region that offers a powerful hand-hold that extends the head on the neck. Patients have told me they get relief from headaches by pressing upward on this region of the medial eye socket, presumably as this extension vector counters a physiological flexion that is part of the headache.
- The meridian then tracks over the head lateral to the midline but it has a deep aspect that also tracks with the midline Governing meridian. As the contralateral Bladder meridian is doing the same thing, they are modelled by the Chinese as decussing left/right over the head. Note that the D/V-CF also has a decussation here as the left olfactory nerve

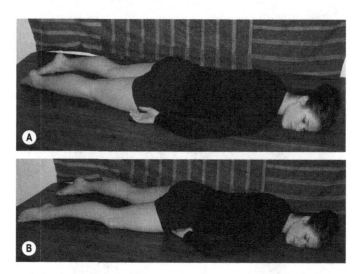

FIG 12.12 **Bladder meridian** This meridian is probably palpated in a prone posture, with the legs both internally and externally rotated.

is primarily left-brain processed, but the left suboccipital muscle is right-brain processed.

- From the vertex of the head, the Bladder meridian drops deep channels to the otic region. Strong para-axial muscles such as the rectus abdominis and the erector spinae power flexion and extension. If this muscular force is not laterally stabilized it will tend to buckle the head on the body. The sternocleidomastoid (SCM) offers that lateral stability to the ventral aspect of the D/V-CF, whist the dorsal aspect is stabilized by the SCM/trapezius, the splenius capitis, and the rectus capitis posterior major. To summarize the effect of these lateral-stabilizing muscles it would be valid to draw lines that course from the vertex to the otic region, as the Chinese meridial map indicates. Power without stability is a dangerous combination.
- The inner Bladder meridian is on the high point of the erector spinae – all of these acupoints extend the spine and are located in the dorsal domain of the D/V-CF. This meridian acts as the para-axial lines of control over the dorsal midline (Du meridian). The meridian is said to wrap around the anus, as expected from an embryological perspective, and also links to the ventral body at the bladder organ. Remember from the embryological chapter that if the ventral migration of the dorsal muscle is inhibited, the bladder organ is left exposed at birth.
- The outer Bladder channel was a necessary addition as an intermediate line of control was needed to initiate extension twists. I do not know when the Chinese theorists split the Bladder meridian but I can understand from a biomechanical perspective why they had to erect a meridian on the rib angles and the lateral raphe of the lumbar region.
- The Bladder meridian continues down the posterior aspect of the leg to the knee. When a patient is prone the normal lie of the legs is to have the heels roll laterally (internal leg rotation). The acupoints on the

posterior knee and calf (Bladder-40/55/56/57/58) reflect hand-holds that would encourage this 'normal' leg position. For example, the Bladder meridian tracks the midline of the calf to Bladder-57, then moves slightly inferiorly and laterally to Bladder-58. When one is prone with the legs straight, heels turned laterally, Bladder-58 is a control point for promoting this lie of the legs. The Chinese seem to have a clear sense of 'normal' and the hand-holds used to encourage movement toward 'normal.'

- From Bladder-58 the meridian sends a deep aspect of itself to the Kidney meridian. From a manual therapy perspective, this makes palpatory sense, as to go on encouraging internal rotation of the leg, the hand-hold must cross the lower calf to the medial border of the leg where the hand-holds continue to the medial ankle region of the Kidney meridian to which it is coupled in TCM theory.

- The lateral foot bones are derived from the dorsal aspect of the developing limb bud. The Chinese take the Bladder meridian, a Yang/ dorsal meridian to the lateral foot. From a manual analysis of the ankle/ foot acupoints I suspect the Chinese used two positions of the legs to map acupoints on this channel. The first position is with the patient prone, legs straight, and with heels falling laterally, as described above. If the legs are abducted when the patient is prone it is then normal for the legs to externally rotate. In this legs abducted, externally rotated posture the lateral foot acupoints are available for palpation. Most people prefer, or are more comfortable in, one or other of these leg postures. Access to both leg postures is the ideal.

KIDNEY MERIDIAN

- The Kidney meridian is analogous to the Heart meridian of the arm. The leg portion of this meridian tracks the ventral post-axial border. Most texts depict this meridian as starting on the sole of the foot in a depression between the second and third metatarsals. However, as predicted by this decoding hypothesis, the meridian sends a deep channel to beneath the little toe. Note that there are few acupoints on the feet, as needles would need to be thick and sharp to penetrate the sole of the foot.

- The posture shown in Figure 12.13 exposes the acupoints to palpation. Note how there is no 'bite' to a line of palpation from the knee to the groin in this posture. The soft tissue absorbs the pressure with little pain – hence no acupoints.

- The Kidney meridian acts on the torso as para-axial lines of control over the ventral midline. From the leg, the meridian is said to touch the tip of the coccyx, then continues via a deep extension to the pubis where it is said to emerge. Just above the pubis, the meridian sends a deep channel to the midline thus allowing the meridian to left/right decuss in the low abdomen.

- Nabil Rizk, in his description of the abdominal wall, describes lines just lateral to the linea alba (Rizk 1980): the Kidney meridian tracks those lines.

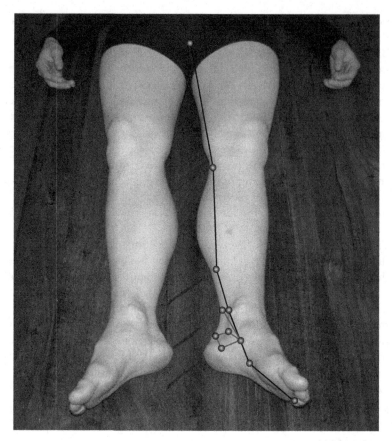

FIG 12.13   Kidney meridian The meridian is internally/externally related to the Bladder
meridian, and probably palpated in the supine posture. It begins beneath the
little toe.

- The Kidney meridian then tracks the V-CF by placing acupoints in the interchondral spaces lateral to the sternum.
- The V-CF courses up from the parasternal interchondral muscles to the root of the tongue. Two thousand years ago, the Chinese drew a deep meridian to the root of the tongue. Was this an accident or insight?

STOMACH MERIDIAN

- The Stomach and Spleen meridians act together to control the pre-axial border of the lower limb. On the torso, both meridians are placed on the intermediate abdominal wall so both initiate twisting movements and, accordingly, from a CF perspective, they track helical biodynamics. Hence the Chinese seem to be linking the leading edge of the lower limb to helical biodynamics of the torso.
- The Stomach meridian starts between the eyeball and the infraorbital ridge. The CF model embeds the eyes at the apex of helical movement patterns. I was drawn to the embedding of sense organs in CFs by this

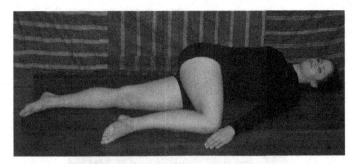

FIG 12.14 **Stomach meridian** There is a spinal twist to expose the meridian. Note the twist exposes the nipple line, and with the arm internally rotated with the head turned up, many of the acupoints are available for palpation.

meridian and its unequivocal linking of intermediate lines of control on the torso to the intermediate sense organ, the eye. The Stomach meridian then tracks the infraorbital foramina and in a straight line continues to the lateral margin of the mouth, Stomach-4. This acupoint sits astride a structure called the modiolus that is a compact, dense, mobile, fibromuscular mass that nine muscles converge on, spiralize into, and reradiate from, with astounding complexity (Williams 1995). The two modioli are a similar structure to the perineal body of the pelvic floor. If you use your index finger and thumb you can palpate the modiolus as a thickening at the corner of the mouth. The early Chinese acupuncturists seem to have a knack for discerning biodynamic nodal regions.

- The Stomach meridian meets the midline above and below the mouth, just inside the hairline of the scalp, below C7 of the spine, in the region of the stomach, and then in a broad midline region from the navel to the pubis. Also on the torso, the meridian tracks to the eye and nipple, structures that I locate in the H-CF. Here we have a meridian that has all the hallmarks of a comprehensively decussed function. This meridian is all about twisting – the Chinese link that biodynamic to the stomach organ.
- Figure 12.14 demonstrates the type of posture that was used in the mapping of the Stomach and Spleen meridians. When the leg is resistant to internal rotation, many of the hand-holds that give leverage for the twist become painful.
- All of the acupoints on the leg are hand-holds that internally rotate the leg. As the practitioner internally rotates the straight leg of a supine patient with a thumb applied to Stomach-36, then 37, 38, and 39, the hand-holds approach the crest of the tibia to a point where it is crossed, and therefore the purchase for the hand-hold is lost. The Chinese just started another line of hand-holds by backing up to Stomach-40, and then moving down the leg with Stomach-41/42/43/44, and finally the lateral nail point of the second toe, Stomach-45. The meridian here is a classic example of the hand-hold methodology employed by the Chinese to map a manual reality that I confirm in my practice every day. As the decoding model would predict, the Chinese have run a deep meridian to

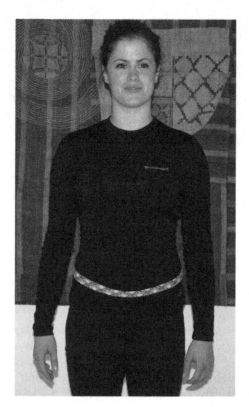

FIG 12.15   The Girdling (or Dai Mai) meridian

the big toe at Spleen-1. Applying too much internal rotation pressure to the big toe would only stress the metatarso-phalangeal joint – they found it more manually effective to track to the second toe but acknowledge the theory via the deep meridian to the big toe.

GIRDLING MERIDIAN (DAI MAI MERIDIAN)

- It is like a loose belt that encircles the lower torso. It is said to bind the 12 + 2 meridians that it crosses. From a CF perspective this meridian represents the R-CF. Squeezing the chest wall and diaphragm would compromise respiration so the Chinese did not envisage a Dai Mai above the waist. Likewise a squeezing of the torso inferior to the iliac crest will not affect body diameter as the sacroiliac joints are very robust.
- The Dai Mai meridian crosses the ventral midline in the region of Ren-6 to Ren-4. This region is given special significance in Chinese culture. The Dantian (or Cinnabar field, or Hara) is where the deepest energies reside and is the source of all movement. I remember, as a student of aikido, the teacher imploring us to move from the Hara, but I had little sense of why. From a CF perspective this is also a special region of profound

biodynamic interplay. The dorsal and ventral domains of the D/V-CF seamlessly fuse below the navel. The L-CF also has a pivot here as left/right movements above the lower abdomen are constrained by the ribs, and below the lower abdomen the ilia are too strongly braced to allow side-bending. The H-CF courses to insert on the inguinal ligaments from the contralateral sides of the body-wall so that they cross below the navel creating the human waist that is so important for our gait pattern which is derived from a contra-rotation of the upper and lower girdles. Importantly, the R-CF has a powerful compressive effect in the lower abdomen as the rectus abdominis dives deep to the fascia of the obliques and the transversus abdominis. I demonstrate the value of this compressive effect to my patients with a new tube of toothpaste that I kink in the top third of the tube. Squeezing the middle of the tube (the solar plexus) will only partially de-kink the tube but also will concurrently risk rupturing the lower seal. Squeezing the bottom of the toothpaste tube protects the lower seal and drives the gel up the tube to de-kink it. Our bipedal stance necessitated a strengthening of the pelvic floor that was allied with a mechanism for generating visceral lift. Also, the kidneys are associated with a loin-to-groin pattern of pain distribution. As half of your body weight is above this lower abdominal region and half below, I now can understand why the lower abdomen was singled out for such special consideration regarding movement, both internal and external.

SUMMARY

The meridial web did have a weaver, many weavers in fact. With a tradition of manual therapy allied with bloodletting and cauterization practices, the ancients, using a whole-organism paradigm, began the mapping and encoding of their insight. They thought long and hard about the nature of movement and how to control it.

A new model of human movement, the contractile field (CF), facilitates the biomechanical understanding of whole-organism movement patterns. Defining field borders and looking for nodal regions where fields of contractility meet and change direction facilitates an enquiry that is congruous with many aspects of the Chinese meridial map. Lines emerge on the living body that will initiate a similar recoil vector and this has been illustrated using a thought experiment. The notion of 'border control' was introduced as a way of refining the recoil reflex. In essence, it is hypothesized that the Chinese have mapped a minimum number of lines to predictably control subtle human shape, or let us call it 'functional shape.' Traditional acupuncture point prescriptions, from this perspective, are a form of shape manipulation. Shape and function are deeply interdependent.

The Chinese brought expertise from many fields of enquiry to bear on the genesis of the meridial map. Their culture, 2000 years ago, numbering more than 50 million people, was powerful because of the taming of wild rivers that brought wealth, but also too often, catastrophe. They discovered and domesticated rice, the large-scale production of which needed an exquisite control of water. Those large engineering projects needed to be protected from the barbaric outside world so borders became a national obsession (consider the great walls of China). Fluid dynamics and the importance of borders must have been part of the intellectual ethos that was applied to an understanding of the body. The average household would have had babies, toddlers, adults, and the elderly all closely interacting; the developmental cycle, was something they lived with and could muse upon. So a complex mix of an emerging control over water, borders, martial arts, developmental cycles, and the ever-present reality of pain – all factored in the way they mapped an emergent property of the human adult, the most stable of the developmental stages. That insight is still relevant today.

What are the advantages of this approach to understanding the meridial map?

- A methodology available to the Chinese 2000+ years ago
- Suggests why acupuncture is ineffective if the patient is too tired or deficient, and why meridians are not found on the cadaver
- Suggests why meridians are not found on babies
- Models why there are 12 + 2 meridians
- Explains the 'exterior–interior' relationship
- Explains the 'six channels' relationship
- Explains the 'deep' channels
- A hand-hold methodology that follows borders helps understand the location of acupoints
- Aids the understanding of traditional point prescriptions via the manipulation of shape
- Suggests new avenues of enquiry and research
- Suggests the possibility of taking the old medical map into new domains. The author is interested in the application of the meridial map to computer three-dimensional animation where shape control is of great interest. Rather than a joint-based approach to animation, the Chinese have sustained an enquiry into a morphological field-based approach to controlling movement.

The practice of traditional acupuncture in the modern world must prove itself to be clinically and economically effective. Developing an understanding of what the Chinese mapped is an important first step in asking the right research questions of traditional practice. There will be wheat to separate from the chaff but the jury is out as to the size of the sieve.

> *The principal value of myths and rites is to preserve until the present time the remains of methods of observation and reflection which were (and no doubt still are) precisely adapted to discoveries of a certain type: those which nature sanctioned from the starting point of a speculative organization and exploitation of the perceptible world in terms of perception. This science of the concrete was necessarily restricted by its essence to results other than those destined to be achieved by the exact natural sciences, but it was no less scientific and its results no less genuine. Those results, having been affirmed ten thousand years before others, still underpin our own civilization.*

Levi-Strauss 1972

REFERENCES

Blakeslee S, Blakeslee M 2007 The body has a mind of its own: how body maps in your brain help you do (almost) everything better. Random House, New York

Blaschko J 1901 Die Neven-verteilung in der Haut in ihrer Beziehung zu den Enkrankungen der Haut. Beilage zu den Verrhandlungen der Deutschen Dermatologischen Gesellschaft VII Congress, Breslau

Cox P, Balick M 1994 The ethnobotanical approach to drug discovery. Scientific American 270(6):82–87

Deadman P, Al-Khafaji M, with Baker K 1998 A manual of acupuncture. Journal of Chinese Medicine Publications, Hove

Fitzgerald M 1998 The birth of pain. Medical Research Council, Summer, No. 78

Howlett R 1998 Simple minds. New Scientist 2139:29–32

James R 1993 Linear skin rashes and the meridians of acupuncture. European Journal of Oriental Medicine 1(1):42–46

Jing C 1982 Anatomical atlas of Chinese acupuncture points. Shandong Science and Technology Press, Jinan

Kaptchuk T 1983 Chinese medicine; the web that has no weaver. Rider, London

Kingsland J 2000 Border control. New Scientist; Life Sciences 132, Inside Science supplement 15 July

Levi-Strauss C 1972 The savage mind. Oxford University Press, Oxford

Lewis J, Kristan W 1998a Representation of touch location by a population of leech sensory neurons. Journal of Neurophysiology 80:2584–2592

Lewis J, Kristan W 1998b Quantitative analysis of a directed behavior in the medicinal leech: implications for organizing motor output. The Journal of Neuroscience 18(4):1571–1582

Lu Gwei-Djen, Needham J 1980 Celestial lancets; a history and rationale of acupuncture and moxa. Cambridge University Press, Cambridge

Rizk N 1980 A new description of the anterior abdominal wall in man and mammals. Journal of Anatomy 131(3):373–385

Scorzon C 2003 Acumoxa: the role of standardised textbooks in teaching and learning acumoxa in contemporary China. The European Journal of Oriental Medicine 4(2)

Williams P 1995 Gray's anatomy, 38th edn. Churchill Livingstone, Edinburgh

CHAPTER 12 • *Decoding the Chinese meridial map*

185

Manipulating shape

13

*So much contemporary research appears to be misdirected by the lack of a sufficiently
empowered conceptual model that would aid that important first step in any research,
which is to ask the right questions.*

It is time to review and take stock of the ideas introduced in the preceding
chapters. A frame of view was created in the first chapters via two lenses. A
long-range lens was employed to peer back in time to the origin of movement
over half a billion years ago. That lens looked at our phyla, our tribe writ
large, as we are vertebrate. We embody the basic constructional forms
common to all our phyla. Yes, from our perspective we are a special case
because we are bipedal and large brained; however, a massive momentum
yet binds us to the past.

A short-range lens peered into our embryonic morphogenesis, describing,
albeit briefly, a process that we have all lived experientially. Cleaving, com-
pacting, gastrulating, folding – deep in our cellular memory we know these
momentous processes. The genesis of one's basic shape is derived from these
processes that take place within the first 6 weeks post-conception, but shape
continues to change over the course of a lifetime.

Our movement patterns certainly reflect these momentums. Side-bending
is still a primal generator of movement. Each time we take a step we hitch
one side of our pelvis up via the lateral contractile field (L-CF) so the leg can
swing forward. But, like a dolphin, we have also acquired the ability to flex
and extend, here called the dorso/ventro contractile field (D/V-CF). Coupling side-bending with flexion or extension creates a spinal torque that our
species has exploited more than any other, the helical contractile field (H-CF)
that wraps around the body to conceptually emerge at the eyes. We have
employed contra-rotation of the shoulders and pelvis for our bipedal gait and
projectile throwing. Moreover, our lumbar spine has seamlessly blended

187

© 2010 Elsevier Ltd / Inc / Bv
DOI: 10.1016/B978-0-7020-3109-0.00018-3

these movement imperatives together to create a form of spinal gearbox that I described in the chapter on H-CF. The CF model bootstraps muscles together around these primal movements to form large functional fields that interactively are complex enough to describe what we see humans actually do in movement.

Limbs are not just appendages made from muscle and bone. From a CF perspective they emerge from specific sites on the embryonic body-wall that engenders the limb buds with a close affinity to helical biodynamics, here simplified as the limb contractile fields (Limb-CFs). Limbs express and amplify twisting motions generated by the body-wall. Limb function can only be understood with reference to developmental processes that start with the limb bud, continue to the tightly flexed postures of the full-term neonate, to then conform to floor sitting postures and the erection from the floor to standing, walking, and running. A joint-by-joint, muscle-by-muscle analysis of limb function will miss essential insights that the CF perspective will engender. As hands and feet are a primary interface with the environment they are given special significance in the CF model.

We would tend to buckle if our bodies had not developed a protective mechanism. Squeezing the body-wall maintains our longitudinal integrity, a function I call the radial contractile field (R-CF). Core strength is not just the transversus abdominis (TA). To reduce the anti-buckling mechanism of the spine to a single named muscle is ludicrous. Likewise, to describe the musculature as comprising inner and outer units, the so-called inner unit hollowing that stabilizes the abdomen whilst the outer unit moves the body, is a simplification carried too far. As a model of spinal function, the inner unit/ outer unit is an abstraction that detracts from clarity. Rather, spinal stabilization is a whole-body squeeze that can only be understood with reference to the coelom that is the interface between the R-CF and the deepest muscles of the body, i.e. the 'visceral' muscles that pump blood (blood itself is mesodermal) and motivate the visceral organs, here called the chiralic contractile field (C-CF). If the visceral organs are inflamed, or if there is excessively high or low blood pressure, the squeezing and sucking role of the R-CF will be compromised.

The CF model then mimics the embryology to consider the role of the intermediate mesoderm. Intermediate mesoderm is closely associated with the kidneys, the coelom, the ectodermal ring, and the genital/gonad systems. Modelling movement without considering the role of the kidneys' influence on fluid physiology is plainly inadequate from a whole living organism perspective. Our modern, heavily salted and sugared diets are playing havoc with our physiology, which in turn predisposes us to musculoskeletal distress.

WHY ARE CONTRACTILE FIELDS IMPORTANT? HOW MIGHT THEY BE USED IN CLINICAL PRACTICE?

Like a lot of research or modelling, the practical outcomes are often obscure at the onset of the enquiry. Analyzing primal patterns of movement led me to consider how to assess these interactive whole-body patterns of movement – hence the archetypal postures and the concept of biomechanical tune. Tune as a concept is predicated on a vision of whole function. If a mechanic is presented with car parts (pistons, valves, water pump, etc.) the concept of tune is not even on the agenda. Only a whole working vehicle is amenable to tuning. Tune (in this context) is the harmonious interaction of multiple car systems to achieve agreed functions. If a car engine has its output increased then brakes, suspension, chassis strength, etc. all need attention, otherwise the increased engine output will destroy the car. Likewise, too much machine-based exercise that tries to extract a muscle from the whole, allied to the loss of ease in the archetypal postures, leads to biomechanical breakdown. Power and poise are derived from a healthy physique that tunefully integrates primal movement imperatives into whole-body patterns that are our birthright. To assist our patients towards movement ease as a first step we need to reactivate basic self-corrective modalities.

The value of the model is in its generality. Each of the many manual therapies and the exercise prescription professions bring generations of expertise to the table, so each profession will explore different aspects and employments of the CF model. I use the CF model on a daily basis in clinical practice so here I muse on these subjects. These applications are derived from my background in osteopathic soft tissue and manipulative techniques, allied with the TCM application of meridial therapy to acupuncture and manual therapy (tui na).

MANUAL THERAPY

The CF model helps with the interpretation of a case history. What brings the patient to me? Where does it hurt, for how long, how did the hurt start, is the condition steady, improving, or deteriorating, what makes it feel better or worse? Then I set a context by asking for anything that significantly traumatized the patient in each decade of their life. Teeth knocked out, broken noses, eye operations, finger trauma, genital abuse, etc. mark the person in a deep manner. Insults and injuries to sense organs (eyes, ears, nose, teeth, tongue, genitals, hands/feet) are weighted significantly in the case history. Bad eyesight is now commonly corrected via contact lens and laser surgery so there can be no external sign of the visual deficit. Correcting vision is one of our great quality-of-life enhancements, but do consider that the eye organ sits astride whole-organism movement patterns and that beneath the visual correction there will be a deeper pattern of historical musculoskeletal adaptation. Beware when a case history starts to stack up sense organ insults. Beware when nodal regions such as the suboccipital, the linea alba, and the pelvic floor are compromised. Beware when basic physiology is deranged, as evidenced by high or low blood pressure, blood sugar issues, and chronic digestive distress.

Following the case history, I will examine the injured body part using standard orthopedic procedure in an attempt to name the offending tissue. Usually this is not possible with any degree of certainty as most frank pathology ends up at the accident and emergency ward of the local hospital. Most patients present with a mosaic of complaints that defy tissue-causing symptoms diagnosis, with diagnoses such as regional pain becoming common (Taylor et al 2004). Even when modern investigative technology reveals damaged tissue, all too often we find that degree of tissue abnormality in the asymptomatic population (Jensen et al 1994). Having said that, it is important to create for the patient a story that addresses their need to know what is causing their pain.

If it is appropriate (as it usually is), I will assess the archetypal postures. Simply asking the patient to sit on the floor in a variety of postures, and noting their ease or dis-ease as they descend and erect from the floor informs me of the tune of key aspects of their biomechanical lives.

Trigger points (TPs) and their relationship to acupoints are not well understood (see Birch 2003, Dorsher 2008, Melzack et al 1977). Hundreds of TPs have been mapped by Travell and Simons (1993) that are largely referenced back to dysfunction in named muscles, trigger points that are more similar in concept to the Chinese notion of Ah-Shi points which translate as the 'Oh Yes!, that's the right spot' points (Hong 2000). Every manual therapist is familiar with these enigmatic sources of acute pain that emerge when palpated. When talking to a psychotherapist some issues appear to be analogous to TPs in that a fair question such as 'how is your mother' can evoke a heated response or a quick diversion towards another subject. The psyche does not want to explore that issue as it is bundled with distress. Likewise, when a body part is restricted in a particular direction, try palpating for the control points that, when pushed, will move the limb or body part in the restricted direction. Control points are loci on the limb and body-wall that, when pushed, move the body in the required direction. For example, if a patient is supine with one leg flexed at the hip and knee, various points on the lateral thigh, knee, and lateral compartment of the lower leg will adduct the leg with different elements of rotation depending on the point of pressure.

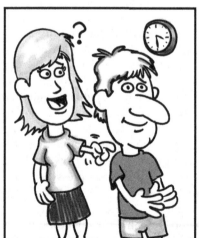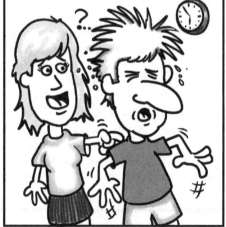

FIG 13.1 This cartoon explores a fair question. What is fair at 15.30 is perceived by the man as unfair at 17.55. Trigger points are mobile entities and react differently as physiological contexts change. *Original drawing by MONSTAcartoons (Mark O'Brian), © Elsevier.*

Acupuncture points have been selected from lines that are discernable from a manual therapy perspective. As discussed in Chapter 12 the acupoints on the Heart and Lung meridians (as examples of the principle) are understandable and reproducible from person to person. That is why they came to be specifically marked and categorized by the Chinese. In contrast, TPs and Ah-Shi points are more nuanced and influenced by many aspects of physiology. As whole-organism tune returns via more floor-based ease, manual or acupuncture treatment of tissue texture, and a diet that is easier on the physiology, many of these trigger points regress.

Manual therapists appear to practice a form of tissue fascism, with each profession specializing in a tissue category. Glibly, the patient is told they have a myofascial problem, or an alignment issue, or a lesion at a specific joint – diagnoses that are too general or too specific. Each group claims to be able to palpate and diagnose tissue that those uninitiated to the practice would find incredulous. For example, manipulative therapists claim to be able to palpate very small derangements in the spinal facet joints or sacroiliac joint, but research does not back up their claims as inter-examiner and intra-examiner reliability is often poor (Panzer 1992). Therapists who work using a cranial motion model claim to palpate movement between cranial sutures, with some even claiming to be able to palpate a restricted first neonatal breath. Acupuncturists claim to be able to palpate the state of one's organs via the radial pulse. For example, when the liver organ is stressed it is claimed that a special area of the radial pulse will take on a wiry feel that is discernable. Each group makes claims that those outside the paradigm would find untenable.

For these reasons I tend to restrict my diagnosis and interpretation to the discernable. When I diagnose a motion restriction it is usually obvious to both the patient and myself. If I palpate a TP the patient can agree with me that that point on the body is unusually tender to palpate. Often I will palpate the contralateral side to demonstrate to the patient the difference in subjective feeling from what I would call a 'fair question' of the tissue. A fair question is important to any examination.

Plucking a guitar string, not too hard or too soft, at the correct location on the string, and listening for the appropriate tone is a normal question asked of that guitar string – it should sound pleasing. When I palpate for TPs I use a pressure and location that are appropriate for that person. A fair question from a manual therapy perspective is a range of movement, or a manual pressure that in health should feel 'normal' for that person, in fact it should feel 'good.' When I get an unusual response I am alerted to work that needs to be done.

The CF model is a stark contrast to the manual paradigm I was taught at osteopathic college. We were required to be able to palpate individual spinal or peripheral joints for motion restriction. Joints acting above and below the site of lesion were also to be assessed. In contrast, the CF model encourages one to palpate far and wide, via a rationale framework, for related areas of a complex mosaic that is neuromusculoskeletal pain.

Two concepts I use in manual therapy treatment will be touched on now. The first is the concept of 'three points of contact.' Many soft tissue techniques can be moderately painful for the patient but, in my experience, patients want the tender areas or TPs accurately located and will tolerate some pain if they think the therapeutic outcome will be improved. Three points of contact is a way of treating a painful area that minimizes the perceived pain felt by the patient.

The practitioner places one hand (the applicator) to work on the TP or sore tissue, one hand supports that body area, and a third point of contact is established via the practitioners' body to create a subtle third point of contact that is reassuring to the patient. The concept is analogous to the positive, negative, and neutral (or ground) of a three-pin electrical socket.

For the first point of contact the practitioner places the fingers or thumbs on the patient's tender area. The pressure applied here can be light or deep, static or gently pulsing. The second hand supports this action by lightly compressing the patient's body towards the applicator hand, thereby creating a manual sense of context for the technique. The third point of contact is usually somewhat distant to the site of the trigger point (ipsilateral or contralateral), applied via the outside of the practitioner's body. The third point of contact is often invisible to the patient until it is removed. Patients will notice the difference as a sense of more support and less pain from the troublesome area. Patients with no training in manual therapy can feel the difference immediately, and prefer the three points of contact technique.

The second concept I call 'spreading.' A site of pain on the patient's body is registered on the sensory cortex as a hot spot. The spreading concept is a way of trying to diffuse the brain's sense of the pain over a wider area. In practice the technique involves holding the site of pain (usually after it has been worked on using the three points of contact), whilst the second hand of the practitioner lightly rubs or holds the patient's body at a distance from the primary source of the patient's pain. This light scanning rub may track the same CF that the source pain is located within, or it may purposefully move contralateral. Holding a source of pain also seems to help the practitioner find related TPs that are part of the matrix that has created or sustains the presenting complaint. Usually I will try to track the spreading to a finger or toe, as these are control points for biodynamics of the entire limb.

Eyal Lederman (2000) and I developed the 'harmonic technique' in the 1990s. It is a manual technique that oscillates body parts via harmonics that the practitioner is able to elicit from the patient's passive body. Each body part relates to the whole via an inherent natural resonant frequency. Rocking as a manual technique has deep roots in basic physiological and psychological needs. It is rhythmic, pulsatile, comforting, hydrating, relaxing, and soothing, as evidenced when you pick up a newborn baby and rock it. Eyal's reference work on the technique discusses its effect on fluid flow through the interstitium (the anatomical space surrounding cells) and the lymph network. The harmonic technique is an important tool in the armamentarium of a manual therapist. The CF model sits easily with this approach to manual therapy.

In short, the manual therapies are a broad medley of professions that bring a wide range of skills to the table. Some schools may develop techniques for specific CFs, or exercise systems that will attempt to target a named CF. There is a link between theory and practice but that link in the messy world of biology is rarely direct or linear.

EXERCISE

Before a musician plays an instrument it must be tuned. Tune comes first and foremost. The concept of tune is crucial to a new understanding of musculoskeletal ease/dis-ease, and our approach to exercise. Enlisting self-corrective mechanisms allows the body to regenerate and re-establish tune between bouts of exercise.

For example, a 32-year-old tri-athlete presented to me complaining of neck and shoulder pain whilst on the bike with a stiffness across her thoracic spine that needed constant micro movement of her back and shoulders to relieve. Her whole right side felt dropped, so much so that she felt she was twisted whilst running. Endurance performance was deteriorating with more aches and pains associated with less training. The case history revealed no history of trauma. On examination of a forward bend with legs straight her fingertips were 20 cm from the floor with a pronounced thoracic kyphosis. Squatting was possible only with her heels 6 cm raised, with the attempt to full squat associated with marked hunching of the shoulders. Sitting cross-legged was uncomfortable with both knees raised. When I asked her to bend forward from this posture, little movement ensued with most of that coming, again, from her thoracic spine further flexing.

Here was a very fit athlete who presented with aches and pains that were non-diagnosable from an orthopedic perspective, at best described as a regional pain syndrome. I explained to her my findings regarding her state of biomechanical tune. In the practice, I have pictures of people from all corners of the globe sitting comfortably in archetypal postures. Patients quickly see the inherent correctness of the approach. We went through each floor posture noting how to progress without stretching joint capsules inappropriately. By this, I mean keep your knees over your second toe when you squat, do not collapse the medial arch of the foot, and do not allow the lateral ankle ligaments to overstretch, as discussed earlier. Keep moving from posture to posture whilst using rolled towels and pillows as necessary. The body wants to drop into these postures – they are known. To place a value on floor sitting was my take-home message to her. In this case, I additionally suggested a series of four exercises that I have developed to stretch the H-CF, exercises that are called the 'Leonardo's' after the man in the circle illustration where Leonardo was exploring bodily proportions.

She came back 3 weeks later. After each exercise session she had spent time on the floor. Her ability to do the miles on her bike had returned, as had her ease in movement between exercise sessions. The thoracic kyphosis was less prominent. At this stage manual therapy on trigger points and joint mobility is more likely to have a lasting effect. I then introduced the erectorcises (20–30 repetitions of each) that gave her more strength so that by week five she was posting good training times again.

Here in Wellington, New Zealand, I refer to personal trainers for more specific therapeutic exercise. Phillip Silverman and Glen Small briefly discuss how they have combined the CF model and the archetypal postures in their work.

Central to any robust understanding is the rigor of the underlying theoretical infrastructure. Indeed, any instability that exists within the foundation will bring into question the entire body of knowledge constructed thereafter. This has been of central concern for the manual therapies, particularly within an ever-evolving era of evidence-based practice, where many have struggled to provide scientific support for clinical practice. In part, this may relate to the ongoing controversy and disagreement surrounding the evolving field of functional anatomy where it appears new thinking is required, and Phillip Beach's work is one bold step in this regard.

Phillip has managed to deconstruct the prevailing stranglehold of morbid cadaver-based anatomical thought, a methodology that has served biomedical science well but has defied many of the realities of manual therapy and physical conditioning that remain scientifically indefinable. As basic engineering would remind us, we need to have a solid understanding of the components and their interaction in any given structure otherwise we are destined for problems. In this respect, much modern theory has been built on research that focuses on pathological populations such as those with back pain (Hodges & Richardson 1996, O'Sullivan et al 1997). Thus, evidence constructed on suboptimal functioning has become the basis of clinical assessment and, in turn, treatment.

Phillip's contractile fields model has reintroduced the anatomy of the living that is reminiscent of Vesalius's early seminal work 'of the fabric of the human body,' published some 500 years ago. Although he was depicting anatomy he did it in such a way that acknowledged the living person, using the metaphor of fabric to engender a continuous integrated functional anatomy. Unfortunately, these central tenets appear to have been lost in translation by subsequent thinkers. Phillip has reintroduced these ideas via the use of systems theory and taking us back to the origin of form and structure via the embryology. As Husserl (2001) stated a century ago, 'we need to go back to the things,' that is, to define knowledge in a way that is true to our methods of assessment. In this regard, embryology and evolutionary biology would seem the likely 'things' for discerning the structural make-up of the body. I have used Phillip's work in two major areas of my life, those being sport and teaching.

Sport

As an athlete, I have received much treatment and advice from Phillip that has largely been based on the contractile fields approach. I have found this invaluable on two accounts, firstly the promotion of physical restoration, and secondly on the assessment of 'biomechanical tune.' Ultimately, it is recovery from training rather than training in its own right that leads to progress. In this regard, Phillip's archetypal floor postures are an ideal strategy for those pursuing athletic endeavors as it is both cost effective and can be done in conjunction with other activities, meaning that it can be easily integrated into any training regime. Many athletes know when training is going well – sessions are easy to perform and require minimal effort. In contrast, the opposite is true when problems occur. In this respect I have found the archetypal postures an effective warning system for potential emerging issues, as a lack of ease in the postures is often indicative of problems to come.

Muscles and meridians

Teaching

Often I am asked what particular muscle is responsible for a given movement. Based on conventional anatomical teaching, this would be a rational question, but it epitomizes the map not being the territory. The topographical rather than functional mindset of the student is clearly illustrated in this example. The predicament affects not only how students and trainers think about exercise, but also prescription, where the structure of many programs, again, reflects isolated named muscles. This has implications for transferability as the trainee may get stronger at a given exercise yet show no improvement in the activity trained for owing to lack of thought for the integration and functional requirements. Phillip's teaching of the students has challenged many commonly held beliefs, and has provoked many to rethink exercise selection and prescription.

GLEN SMALL
STRENGTH AND PHYSICAL CONDITIONER SPECIALIST

The arena of modern exercise conditioning is replete with isolated, sagittal plane exercises, most of which bear little relationship to the integrated, functional patterns that epitomize human movement. Reliance on strength conditioning machines is ever greater and there seems to be a paucity of specialist conditioning coaches to stem the tide of misinformation currently flooding the health and fitness industry.

This misinformation stems from equipment manufacturers, who merely want to sell exercise machines, and from poorly educated graduates of exercise science courses, in which anatomy is taught piecemeal. Students graduate with vague recollections of each individual piece of the jigsaw of the human body, and with poor understanding of movement and function. There is no grasp of the body as an entire organism, a wholly functioning unit of biology, the result of a miraculously complex embryology, which in itself is the summation of millennia of evolution.

What is needed is a change of paradigm. I believe that the contractile fields model is exactly the paradigm shift that is required in the conditioning community. Using Phillip's model, fields of contractility become the cornerstone of exercise prescription. Swathes of interconnected soft tissue and patterns of movement take over from isolated, non-functional muscle-conditioning exercises, as typified in bodybuilding programs, which predominate in gymnasia today. Neuromuscular and musculoskeletal function are enhanced using this model of interconnectivity. Exercise prescription is immediately meaningful, safe, and cohesive, and postures of repose ('retuning of the body') become central to good recovery.

For example, the helical field (rotational movement) is massively under-represented in most gym-based exercise. The power of rotation in the spine of highly evolved human bipeds is seldom harnessed in a typical exercise regime, yet how many human movements entail twisting? In Phillip's own words, 'When human beings get serious, they get twisted.' Think of a javelin thrower, a bowler in cricket, a golfer or tennis player, judogi, or a practitioner of tai chi chuan.

A more integrated, interconnected, cohesive, and truly three-dimensional appreciation of human movement is what is needed in the fitness industry today to condition people in a meaningful, long-term way. The contractile fields model is, in my long experience, the most complete ideation of human function, to the most profound levels, embracing the full 'warp and weft' of the human body. This model has augmented beyond measure my effectiveness as an exercise-conditioning specialist. I believe that all those in the fitness industry would benefit enormously by embracing this model.

WIDER IMPLICATIONS

Tackling our society's endemic musculoskeletal distress needs new thinking. In particular, we need to rethink some of our social norms and work habits. Prolonged chair sitting is detrimental to our well-being. If one's professional life is desk-bound, many hours per day, for many years, it would be prudent to adapt the workplace to bodily norms that have been established over hundreds of generations. Chairs should be only a part-time prop for our work. I suggest we need a floor-to-standing revolution in desk design. Floor-to-standing work stations (Erector desk) need to be designed and trialled.

A desk that lowered far enough for cross-legged or Japanese sitting would be an obvious place to start redesigning the workplace. This is not far fetched. For most of our evolutionary history as tool fabricators and users, we would have worked from the floor. As I have suggested, the floor-based sitting postures are built into our biomechanical design brief. Floor sitting lowers the vertical height venous blood needs to travel to return to the heart. The major blood vessels of the legs follow fascial planes that emerge structurally and functionally when floor sitting. As one posture becomes uncomfortable, there are multiple options to relieve the pressure. With wireless laptops now the norm workstations could be cheaply equipped with cushions and props for staff who felt like an hour (or three) on the floor.

From the low desk position the work height needs to be easily lifted to a normal chair-based height, where we may spend most of our day, or not. A manual or electrical lift, with adequate cable management, would make the transition quick and painless. Chairs need to be able to move with the body so that static stresses on the physique are minimized. Under my desk I have reflexology rollers, as I have found stimulating the feet with sensory information helps concentration.

To then be able to lift the workstation to a standing height offers yet more postural variety for the physique, and that is what it wants – options. In Wellington where I am based we have the Weta Digital animation studios. Animators spend long hours at computers working on their craft. Many of them find standing desks help with their pains. Standing allows a normal lumbar lordosis, and facilitates weight transfers from one leg to the other. If you imagine yourself as a big bag of fluid, tipping the fluid bag initiates a wholesale fluid drive from top to bottom. Productivity will increase when people are freed of the ill-fitting constraints of desk-based life.

A floor-to-standing workstation is the obvious fix to many of our desk-sitting ills. What is needed is a culture change. We now see ourselves as so civilized, the thought of a suited professional sitting cross-legged is slightly ludicrous. Companies that do initiate these workplace interventions will be talked about and studied. People will quickly adapt to the workplace change, some by not changing their habits, others by employing the whole package.

A rock garden walkway in the office environment would be another cost-effective intervention in the battle against chronic musculoskeletal pain. It is a battle we are losing at present, as there has been no easy fix to emerge from the many therapeutic professions that attend it. Walking on a rock pathway from one area of the office or home to another might seem a naïve suggestion, but I can assure you that, after the initial banter had subsided, many people in the office would walk this talk. Bodies are a whole matrix and to cut our feet from the rest of us is placing a handicap on the matrix.

The Western sitting toilet is now the norm in the developed world, yet another of our more dubious cultural exports. To sit at the toilet in the now conventional posture is as functionally handicapping as giving birth trussed up with stirrups.

The erectorcise exercises are made for children. Getting up and down from the floor repeatedly is a natural activity for kids. The exercises are simple, propless, easy to teach, and of lifelong value. Schools are ripe for some of these ideas. Floor sitting should be encouraged when possible. Trying to re-tune a body that has set deeply embedded patterns of discordance is far harder than when young and still establishing basic patterns of musculoskeletal organization.

FUTURE DIRECTIONS

A book such as this has to balance the needs of many different types of audience. The specialist in evolutionary anthropology, embryology, or structural anatomy will need more detail than has been given. But each new word often entails two or three new words to explain it and word count rapidly soars. Many of the professions likely to read a book like this will want more 'how to' examples or prescriptions. I have resisted this as manual technique taught via a book is usually of limited value. One way to judge value in the ideas presented in this book will be to see how the ideas may shape the future direction of research and practice, often in unforeseen directions.

The CF model is amenable to computer modelling, so much so that I suggest the model, when allied to emergent lines of shape control, will aid in creating better animation programs, and further testing and developing the CF model itself. Computer animation for body movement is largely reliant on three-dimensional motion capture and a joint-based approach to movement. A tight suit worn by the actor has many reflective discs that are usually placed on or near the main joints so that when the actor moves, the three-dimensional camera array can capture and digitize the flow of movement. Gollum, the twisted character from the *Lord of the Rings* films, had seven discs to capture his extraordinary spinal movement. Each spinal segment has at least four joints and the intervening intervertebral disc, so seven luminous discs to cover spinal motion is obviously a simplification. The CF model should help in the placement of the discs, and suggests luminous lines on either side of movement borders might add nuance to animation.

How the limbs interact with the torso may be clarified. There is considerable evidence that the Limb-CFs need to have an anterior/posterior component as well as the dorso/ventro component presented in Chapter 7 (Wolpert 2007). In other words, each limb is constructed via a proximo/distal axis (e.g. shoulder to hand), a dorso/ventro axis as described and modelled in this book, and an anterio-posterior domain in its development (e.g. thumb to little finger). To map the limb's interaction with the torso via dorso/ventro and anterior/posterior domains would add complexity to the model that may or may not add to understanding. Likewise, the chiralic-CF (C-CF) and the fluid field (F-F) are first attempts at modelling the role these systems play in our movement. How these ideas may be tested is open to conjecture; however, the very ability to contemplate human movement in these terms is new and clinically applicable. So there is much work to be done. I envisage the modelling of whole-organism movement patterns will rapidly expand and diversify over the next decades.

The archetypal postures and the erectorcises need to be clinically trialled. It would be really interesting to see the staff on a floor of an office block given floor-to-standing tables and educated re their use. If positive results emerged, would society accept (and appropriately clothe) people sitting on the floor to work?

The practice of acupuncture is bifurcating. There are those who have invested considerable time, effort, and money into absorbing traditional theory and practice. There are those who take shorter courses and who appear to cherry-pick the most clinically effective evidence-based procedures, and dispense with traditional concepts. Both groups claim the moral high ground. There are now many colleges in the Western world that offer degree courses in acupuncture and TCM, so dialogue is vital. Seeing meridians as emergent lines of shape control will help understand the thought processes that informed the genesis of the map, but this does not, per se, argue for the practice. Over the millennia, layer on layer of needless dogma has obscured the manual roots of the profession. The next generation of acupuncturists will hopefully marry the best of both the East and the West to yet again recreate this old practice. Less dogma, but more understanding is required. Our patients deserve nothing less.

REFERENCES

Birch S 2003 Trigger point – acupuncture point correlations revisited. Journal of Alternative and Complementary Medicine 9(1):91–103 (Review)

Dorsher PT 2008 Can classical acupuncture points and trigger points be compared in the treatment of pain disorders? Birch's analysis revisited. Journal of Alternative and Complementary Medicine 14(4):353–359

Hodges PW, Richardson CA 1996 Inefficient muscular stabilization of the lumbar spine associated with low back pain. A motor control evaluation of transversus abdominis. Spine 21(22):2640–2650

Hong C-Z 2000 Myofascial trigger points: pathophysiology and correlation with acupuncture points. Acupuncture in Medicine 18(1)

Husserl E 2001 Logical investigations: volume one. Routledge, London

Jensen M, Brant-Zawadzki M, Obuchowski N et al 1994 Magnetic resonance imaging of the lumbar spine in people without back pain. New England Journal of Medicine 331(2):69–73

Lederman E 2000 Harmonic technique. Churchill Livingstone, London

Melzack R, Stillwell D, Fox E 1977 Trigger points and acupuncture points for pain: correlations and implications. Pain 3(1):3–23 (Review)

O'Sullivan PB, Phyty GD, Twomey LT, Allison GT 1997 Evaluation of specific stabilizing exercises in the treatment of chronic low back pain with radiographic diagnosis of spondylolysis or spondylolisthesis. Spine 22(24):2959–2967

Panzer DM 1992 The reliability of lumbar motion palpation. Journal of Manipulative Physiological Therapeutics 15(8):518–524

Taylor W, Smeets L, Hall J, McPherson K 2004 The burden of rheumatic disorders in general practice: consultation rates for rheumatic disease and the relationship to age, ethnicity, and small-area deprivation. The New Zealand Medical Journal 117(1203):U1098

Travell J, Simons D 1993 Myofascial pain and dysfunction: the trigger point manual. Vols 1 and 2. Lippincott Williams & Wilkins, Philadelphia

Wolpert L 2007 Principles of development, 3rd edn. Oxford University Press, Oxford

Abbreviations and glossary

CONTRACTILE FIELD ABBREVIATIONS (CFs)

C-CF   chiralic contractile field (with pulsatile and peristaltic domains)
D-CF   dorsal domain of the D/V contractile field
D/V-CF   dorso/ventro contractile field
F-F   fluid field
H-CF   helical contractile field
L-CF   lateral contractile field
Limb-CFs   limb contractile fields (with dorsal and ventral moieties)
R-CF   radial contractile field
V-CF   ventral contractile field

GLOSSARY

acoelomate an animal without a coelom

amniotic cavity a cavity between the amnion that is an extra-embryonic membrane, and the embryo proper that is found in birds, reptiles, and mammals. The cavity is filled with amniotic fluid that is nourishing and protecting to the embryo that drinks it, inhales/exhales it, and urinates into it

apical ectodermal ridge (AER) a beautiful linear crest that is a thickening of the ectoderm at the distal end of the bird and mammalian limb bud. It is an extrusion of the embryo encircling ectodermal ring, and is vital to normal limb development

aponeurosis a white, shining membrane that is a sheet-like tendon of a muscle

archetype the original pattern, form, or idealized version of a thing or an animal

body-plan, also known as Baupläne the essential constructional traits that combine to give form, shape, and function to animal life

bradycardia heart slowness, usually fewer than 60 beats per minute for an adult, but endurance training will lower this average

caudal toward the tail end of an animal

cephalic toward the brain end of an animal

chiral a form that is not superposable on its mirror image, e.g. the hands

chordate all the animals that exhibit a notochord at some stage in their life cycle

cloaca the most posterior part of the embryonic hindgut. Placental mammals have separate urinogenital and anal openings

coelom a fluid-filled cavity that forms within the mesodermal layer of triploblastic animals. It partially separates the muscles of the body-wall from the muscles of the gastrointestinal tract. In many animals the coelom acts to collect physiological excretions, and plays a role in the maturation of the gametes (sex cells)

contralateral the opposite side of the body

Dantian the elixir field, a site of real importance in many oriental traditions where it plays a role in meditative and martial arts. It is usually located about three finger widths below the navel and deep to the skin

decuss to cross

diploblastic a body-plan that has two (ectoderm/endoderm) embryonic layers that are separated by a gelatinous material

ectoderm the outer layer of a triploblastic body-plan. It forms skin and most of the

201

nervous system, and the most anterior and posterior portions of the digestive tract

ectodermal ring, also known as the Wolffian ridge (as distinct from the Wolffian duct which is an aspect of urogenital development), is a transient ring of thickened epithelium that encircles the 4- to 5-week-old embryo

endoderm in a triploblastic animal it is the innermost cell layer that forms the gut lining

epaxial situated on the dorsal side of an axis

epiblast the outermost layer of an embryo before it differentiates into the definitive mesoderm and ectoderm

epimere a term used in comparative anatomy meaning the paraxial meso-derm on the dorsum of the animal, in vertebrates the segmented somites

gastrulation following the cleavage period the embryo undergoes enormous morphological transformation during which the vertebrate body-plan is laid down

haemocoel a body cavity that contains blood. It is not a coelom but plays a role in fluid circulation and may act as a hydrostatic skeleton

holoblastic cleavage a form of cleavage that is found in zygotes with relatively little yolk so the cleavage furrow extends through the entire egg to produce cells of roughly equal size

homology a 'sameness' in structure or morphology due to common ancestry

hydrostat a muscular hydrostat is similar in function to a hydrostatic skeleton except there is no fluid-filled cavity. The entire structure is muscle that can coherently change shape but not volume. It is used to move the body or manipulate items, e.g. the tongue

hypaxial lying ventral or beneath the vertebral axis

hypoblast used in comparative anatomy where it usually refers to the endoderm layer of the embryo

hypomere used in comparative anatomy to refer to the lateral plate, which is the lateral or ventral portion of the mesoderm that contains the coelomic cavity

hypotonic used in physiology when one solution contains a lower concentration of impermeable solutes than intracellu-lar fluid

induction used in embryology to describe how one tissue causes an adjacent tissue to differentiate in a particular way

invaginate to double back within itself

involution a rolling or curling inwards, a retrograde reduction in form and function

ipsilateral on the same side

isotonic a cellular environment where an equal concentration exists both inside and outside a cell

lateral plate mesoderm in vertebrate embryos this mesoderm is lateral and ventral to the somites, and gives rise to the tissues of the heart, kidneys, gonads, and blood

mediastinum lies between the sternum and the vertebral column, and includes all the thoracic viscera except the lungs

meroblastic cleavage partial cleavage, usually found in yolk-rich eggs such as found in many fishes, reptiles, and birds

mesoderm the middle layer of triploblas-tic animals, within which the coelom will form. Mesoderm-derived tissues include muscles, bones, tendons, blood/heart, visceral muscle, and much of the urogenital system

mesonephros the middle of the three embryonic kidneys. In aquatic verte-brates it is the main excretory organ; in mammals it has only a temporary excretory function but in males it is appropriated to contribute to the genital system

metanephros the adult kidney that develops from the caudal part of the embryonic nephric ridge

microvilla minute hair-like projections that increase cell surface area

modiolus describes a small, dense chiasma of facial muscles that is just lateral to the mouth. Eight muscles converge to spiralize into the modiolus

moieties halves

morphogenesis the coordinated process of bringing about shape and form to the embryo

morphogenic field a field of activity where changes in form take place

morula refers to the small ball of cells (10–12) that have cleaved from the fertilized egg, before fluid cavities form within

myomere a muscle segment

myosepta the connective tissue that separates myomeres

nephrogenic developing or originating in the kidneys

notochord a defining characteristic of all vertebrates is a cartilaginous rod that is ventral to the spinal cord, about which the vertebral system will form

ontogeny the study of the developmental sequence from the fertilized ovum to maturity

organogenesis the genesis of organs from the ectoderm, mesoderm, and endoderm

osmosis the diffusion of water across a semi-permeable membrane. Net movement is from the less concentrated (hypotonic) to the more concentrated (hypertonic) solution

phylotypic Ernst Haeckel (1834–1919), a German biologist, developed a controversial recapitulation theory (ontogeny recapitulates phylogeny) that suggests all vertebrates share a similar external form in early embryological development, the phylotypic stage. He overstated and probably doctored his early drawings to back his claims up but nevertheless, at this stage in vertebrate development, there exists a commonality between all vertebrates

placode a thickened disc of ectoderm on the embryonic surface that is the first external manifestation of the primary sense organs and some nerves

pronephros the first and most primitive of the three urogenital excretory organs. It is a paired organ that develops from the intermediate mesoderm. In humans it is a transient structure but nevertheless, it is a vital precursor to the correct development of the definitive urogenital system that follows

pulsatile that which pulsates, e.g. the heart

rostral towards the region of the nose and mouth

sensory capsule during embryogenesis the primary sense organs manifest as discrete capsules of development

septum transversum the connective tissue, originating in the upper neck, that will form the central tendon of the diaphragm and much of the muscular component

somite vertebrate development is characterized by whorls of mesoderm that form the segments that lie on the two sides of the neural tube. Different compartments of the somite will contribute to the spine, the muscles of the body, and the skin

somitomeres loose whorls of mesodermal tissue that number about 50 pairs. They are the earliest manifestation of the embryonic process that will form the muscles of the face, jaw, and throat, followed by a caudal progression of somites that will contribute form to the torso of the embryo

splanchnic descriptive of structures that supply the gut. In embryology the splanchnic layer of the lateral plate mesoderm forms the circulatory system and the future gut wall

teratogenic the study of the abnormalities of development

totipotent cells that have total potential. They are able to differentiate into any of the differentiated cells of an organism. Only cells from the first couple of cleavage cycles are thought to retain totipotency. Thereafter, cells may be pluripotent (cells that can give rise to most but not all tissues) or multipotent (cells that can differentiate along only some pathways)

trilaminar disc during gastrulation the bilaminar disc invaginates to form a mesodermal layer to thus become a trilaminar disc

triploblastic an animal with three germ layers: ectoderm, mesoderm, endoderm

ureteric buds at the caudal end of the Wolffian duct the ureteric buds sprout. These will form the ureters and much of the plumbing of the definitive kidneys but not the nephrons

Wolffian duct, also known as the mesonephric duct Caspar F Wolff, a German physiologist (1733–1794), discovered the primitive kidneys (mesonephros) and the ducts that connect them to the cloaca. These ducts degenerate in the female but in the male they differentiate under the influence of testosterone into a series of organs between the testis and the prostate

zygote the fertilized egg

INDEX

Note: the suffixes f, t and b are used throughout for figures, tables and boxes.

Index